This story is dedicated to Wolfgang Lutz (1913–2010), pioneering doctor, whose friendship over 15 years was at once stimulating and challenging, and whose medical insights changed my life in unexpected ways.

Uncle Wolfi's Secret

Valerie Bracken

JUST PERHAPS?

First published in Great Britain in 2013 by

Just Perhaps?

www.justperhaps.co.uk

ISBN 978-0-9926944-0-1

A catalogue record for this book is available
from the British Library

Typeset and designed by Zebedee Design

Printed in Great Britain by
Bell & Bain Ltd, Glasgow

CONTENTS

CONTENTS

PART I

BY THE POND

I have always been fond of my 'Uncle Wolfi'. Ever busy at some idea of his, he was still always ready to stop for a chat. We used to laugh when he came to visit us in England: every time we offered him a plate of chips with his fish, he would say: "Thank you very much, I'll have two." But Uncle Wolfi meant two chips, not two platefuls.

The best times were in the holidays. Uncle Wolfi has been a doctor for many, many years. When he was nearly 80 years old, he retired but soon started to work again. I remember Mum saying that he was not the sort to retire while there was still so much important work to be done. But, luckily for me, in the spring and summer he always spent time in his home in the mountains of Austria. Uncle Wolfi had a big house next to a lake and it is there that I spent so many memorable school holidays playing in his rambling old garden, a garden which had a large pond and an orchard, as well as every bush and plant imaginable.

He has always done a lot of thinking, has Uncle Wolfi. During these holidays, I often used to find him sitting by the huge pond in his garden. Sometimes I would see him staring into the water and at other times he would sit there quietly, shaking his head slowly and frowning. One day I asked him why he shook his head and frowned. He looked up and smiled at my question. Uncle did get grumpy at times, but on the whole he was a kindly old man and I liked him a lot. He paused for a while and then he said softly: "Oh, Sparrow, they just don't see!" Uncle Wolfi often called me ' Sparrow' and it had become my nickname.

"Who don't?" I wondered.

"Oh they – the scientists, the medics, the journalists – more or less all of them," he muttered. "They just don't see," he repeated, looking again into the water.

"Don't see what, Uncle Wolfi?" I pursued eagerly. Then he said something extraordinary.

"They don't see the importance of beginnings." Uncle Wolfi was again shaking his head and frowning. "They don't see who or what we are, because they forget who and what we were – and how on earth can they possibly know what we need, if they don't see who we are!" I didn't have a clue what he was talking about. Here, Uncle Wolfi caught hold of his frowns and tossed them away. Turning to me, he continued more amicably, "Well, let's put it this way – and I don't think I am wrong in this – if we overlook the little we do know about our beginnings, then there is no adequate anchorage for our reasoning which, of course, soon goes adrift. Yes, maybe that's it." I was still mystified.

Then Uncle remained thoughtful for what seemed like a long time. His eyes had a faraway look as he resumed speaking. "It may seem very strange to you but, sometimes, when I look into my pond, it is as if I see right back to the beginning of time." He said this so quietly and with such an air of mystery that I have been asking questions and listening to his stories ever since! For I soon realised that

Uncle Wolfi really did take notice of a bit of history that other people had forgotten, that he knew both important secrets and the origin of some of the secrets. I longed to know more.

Next time I saw him by the pond, I ventured to ask what he saw as he gazed into the water. He didn't answer for many minutes. He just went on gazing. At length he said, in a voice that seemed somehow changed, "I see a time when there was no land on this planet of ours we call earth – a time when all was ocean, when the earth's atmosphere had little oxygen and almost the only living things in existence were tiny organisms with only one cell . . ."

"But how could they breathe with so little oxygen?" I asked, interrupting his reverie. We had done oxygen at school. Uncle blinked a few times before answering.

"Oh, they didn't, not in the way you mean. They fermented rather than breathed."

"Like turning into alcohol?" I asked.

Uncle sighed. "No, more like the sort of fermenting that happens when we salt cabbage and weigh it down with a large stone to make sauerkraut."

"Yuk! Oh, how it must have smelled!"

Uncle made no comment, but sat silent for a while, turning his eyes once more to the pond.

"But to continue. I was talking about the days when there was just ocean and these tiny organisms with one cell were living and multiplying by dividing and fermenting in this 'primordial soup' as they call it." And here he began to chuckle as if at a private joke.

"But what sort of soup was it, Uncle?" I asked intrigued.

My favourite was tomato, or maybe burnt onion, or just perhaps mother's homemade oxtail.

"But that's just it!" exclaimed Uncle, still chuckling but not making any sense that I could see.

Without further explanation, he asked, "Do you know how long ago that was? More than two billion years!" he said, answering his own question. "That means that though I personally have been on this earth a mere 80 years or so, there is a sense in which I stretch back over two billion years!" His eyes twinkled as he looked at my doubting and uncomprehending face. "Oh, there is a sense in which you stretch back that far, too," he said, laughing. "Your father and mother had a father and mother, who had a father and mother, who had a father and mother and so on back and back in time. And then back in time further still, through different ancestral species right back and then back again to the one-celled creatures, then even before that to the very beginning of life on earth."

"When we were all swimming in seafood soup?" I asked hopefully, recalling the bouillabaisse I had once eaten on another holiday.

"Oh little one, be serious for a moment!" But then, remembering I knew nothing of those ancient days, he added: "The time I am talking about was a long, long time before there was anything so complicated as a fish."

He paused awhile, tossing a pebble into the pond. 'You know, even in our present lifetime, we too start out in life as only one cell – one fertilised egg cell from our mother. Fortunately, we progress a little more rapidly: it may have taken something like two billion years for the human species to evolve from one-cell organisms, but now we <u>are</u> human, it only takes around nine months for us to go from one cell to a fully-formed baby with trillions of cells and ready to be born. Amazing, isn't it! I'll tell you all about it one day," he promised. "Well, about some of it anyway."

"Trillions of calls," I repeated, awestruck.

"For now," he added, "just remember that there is always a sense in which we come out of what has gone before and, just as important, that there is always change along the way."

Then we went off together to gather raspberries and I felt a lot easier. Old people say some strange things.

APES

In Uncle Wolfi's garden, I used to play wonderful games. There were mountains all round, which you could see if you stood up. But if I crouched down in the grass, the trees and bushes surrounded me like a tropical forest, and I would imagine wild animals coming to take a drink in the large lake nearby. Instantly I was an ape in the Africa of old, loping along the ground with other apes and emitting little grunting noises. Then I would climb contentedly into one of the gnarled old fruit trees in the search for food.

I remember playing this game towards the end of one summer holiday. I think I was about eight years old at the time. I was sitting in a tree as Uncle Wolfi came by on his regular half-hour walk and I scrambled down to join him.

"Up to monkey business again, I see," he said, winking.

"I am playing ancestral relatives, actually," I replied a little stiffly. "I am not a little monkey as mother would have it. I am a great ape!" I announced proudly.

"Our ape-like ancestors lived millions of years ago," Uncle informed me. "And a lot has happened to us since! They say that the modern chimpanzee developed from a shared ancestry with us, way back when," continued Uncle Wolfi.

"Well, they still feel like our relatives," I said, remembering my visits to London Zoo.

"Then, may I perhaps have the pleasure of addressing you as my little chimp?" he added with a slight bow of his head, but his eyes were laughing.

"All right, Uncle," I agreed cheerfully. "Then I can be a chimp up your tree!" I said, scrambling up again onto a branch to go on with my game.

"Uncle Wolfi," I called out as he was walking away, "I could have my tea up here. Please can I? I know chimps eat fruit, and Aunt Helen has some oranges in the fruit bowl." He stopped, turned round and came back.

"Of course you can. It is certainly better than having your roving chimp friends stripping the leaves and fruit from every tree in sight! I will, I think, also provide some insects and a small mammal to make your tea more authentic," chuckled the big man at the foot of the tree.

"Oh, don't be revolting, Uncle. Anyway, I thought chimps just ate fruit."

"Only most of the time, but also leaves, shoots and roots, so I'll bring you some salad too – I'm afraid that is as close as we can get to the plant food of an equatorial forest – and a little meat for good measure."

"And bread and butter?" I queried.

"Let me see," teased Uncle Wolfi, "now bread comes from wheat, which is a grass seed, and grass seed is hardly the type of food that chimps eat! Anyway chimps haven't learnt to cook. As for butter, no, sorry, and you'll have to pass on the ice cream, too!"

So that is how I got my chimp tea up a tree: an orange,

some salad and a bit of ham, and it didn't seem so very different from what the grown-ups were eating indoors round the table. But then, I still had a lot to learn.

Next morning at breakfast, I found a little heap of bean sprouts by my plate.

"But . . . " I protested, eyeing the cornflakes hopefully – I knew they had been bought in especially for me. But Uncle shook his head. "A glass of milk?" Uncle shook his head again. The smell of the bacon and eggs that the others were eating made my mouth water and Uncle read my longing.

"Come on, play the game, my little chimp," said Uncle encouragingly. "If bean sprouts are not to your liking, you can run along and find some gooseberries in the garden."

"Cream and sugar to go with them?" I asked, making one last try. Uncle looked at me with his head on one side.

"Personally I have no knowledge of chimpanzees milking cows, nor of buying groceries for that matter. Run along now. If you are lucky, you might also find an apple that is already ripe or some late raspberries."

Apart from a few gooseberries, I was not lucky. All I found were some rather hard, greenish and unappetising blackberries. By lunchtime, I was getting decidedly hungry. I sat in a huff, pulling gooseberry prickles out of my fingers and looking disconsolately at my plate of crudités, whilst the family enjoyed braune Kraftsuppe, a brown meat soup that smelled of oxtail and reminded me of home. I toyed with a carrot stick, while Aunt Helen and Uncle Wolfi tucked into roast chicken and mushrooms. Sensing that my tears were not far away, Uncle pushed his plate towards me. Gratefully, I took a chicken leg. After that, I helped myself to two rather large helpings of Schokoladensoufflé, a wonderful pudding made from eggs and dark chocolate with morello cherries on top, not very sweet but infinitely delicious. At this, Uncle raised one eyebrow.

"Meet me by the pond," was all he said.

Later that afternoon, I went down to the pond and Uncle was all smiles. But I wasn't smiling: "You said there is always a sense in which we come out of what went before," I grumbled. "Well, I didn't find it much fun being a chimp. I'd have given a lot for a piece of toast and a hot drink. I was starving! And how was I supposed to enjoy bean sprouts when you were all eating a proper breakfast?" I asked fretfully. Uncle merely raised one eyebrow. "I enjoyed the chicken," I conceded earnestly, "and the pudding was heavenly! Thank you, Uncle Wolfi." Uncle nodded. I know he has a soft spot for Aunt Helen's puddings.

"So, what did you learn, I wonder?" he enquired. I thought about this for a moment.

"I think chimps would go hungry living up here in Austria!"

"Not quite the tropical forest of your imagination then?" asked Uncle. He didn't have to rub it in, did he! "And have you thought what a chimp would eat in winter?" I thought about this too, about the cold and the snow of the mountains and it made me shudder just thinking about it. In fact, I was just deciding I would have to invent fire, when Uncle asked: "Do you still want to be a chimp, my little ancestral relative?"

"I think," I answered slowly, "I would have to become a hunter to survive the winter or maybe a shepherd and drive my sheep down to the valleys when it got colder." I was also picturing a house with a warm fire in the daytime and a warm bed to sleep in at night, rather than a frosty platform of twigs on the branches of a tree.

"So, living in this climate, will you settle for being human after all, do you think?" he asked, watching my face intently.

"I think so, Uncle Wolfi. I really do think so."

"Well, it sounds to me like you've moved on a few million years in one swift bit of realism about your surroundings! You see, we were never really apes, as such! We may have had ancestors in common some four to seven million years ago, but the apes went one way, and we went ours. Separate paths, if you like. Gradually adapting to changes in their circumstances, the gorilla eventually became a gorilla, the chimp a chimp, but they never became human. We humans had our own subsequent history." Then Uncle Wolfi said something I didn't really understand until many years later: "My advice to you, niece of mine, is very simple: never forget you <u>are</u> a human being and not a chimp!"

THE SECRET

The following summer, I was back at Uncle Wolfi's. One day, while we were cleaning up the pond together, I began thinking about all those patients Uncle had got well again. Mum said there were many thousands of grateful people whom Uncle Wolfi had helped.

"How do you do it, Uncle Wolfi?" I asked all of a sudden. "How do I clean ponds?" asked Uncle, raising his head and looking at me, frowning a little.

"No, no, Uncle. How do you get so many people well that have so many horrid things wrong with them? Is it a secret or can you tell me?" I wondered aloud. Uncle Wolfi now burst into laughter.

"A secret, bless my soul, what next!" he said, continuing to chuckle. "Oh little one, my secret is as old as the hills – well almost!" he added as an afterthought. Then he looked at me for a long time as if weighing something up.

"If you really want to know, I'm only too happy to share my 'secret'. It's a nice day. What do you say, Sparrow, to taking out the boat?"

That was a wonderful idea. Uncle Wolfi had a rowing boat and I liked nothing better than sitting dangling my fingers in the water while Uncle rowed across the lake with his strong hands on the oars. It looked so easy when he did it!

So we went to the lake and I clambered in. Uncle pushed us off and rowed us smoothly into the centre of the lake, then put up his oars. From here, we had a good view of the mountains all around. A bird swooped low over the water, then suddenly dipped down, catching a fish in its beak and flew off, still holding tight the wriggling fish. A dragonfly hovered and then darted after its prey.

"Those creatures certainly know what they want for their dinner," Uncle Wolfi mused.

"Of course they do," said I.

"Quite so, of course they do," echoed Uncle smiling. He sat awhile gazing up at the hills.

"Have you ever wondered why dragonflies and birds know what to eat and we humans get ourselves in such a muddle? Such a muddle that you even have lessons at school as to what you ought to want to put in your mouth? Does that not strike you as strange?" I must admit I had not thought about it quite like that.

"But Uncle, what about your secret?" I asked impatiently.

"Hush, child. Slowly, slowly! Some secrets, especially such very old secrets have to be discovered by each person anew. So perhaps I should start by putting a question to you. We are sitting here in a rowing boat. Now, if this boat were a motorboat, would it matter what fuel we put in the engine?"

"Of course it would, silly!" Uncle raised his eyebrows a little at the appellation 'silly', but continued unabashed.

"And if we put in the wrong fuel?" I pulled a face of vague apprehension. "Quite!" said Uncle, nodding in approval. "Now, remember I told you that there are not billions but trillions of cells in our bodies? I bet you didn't know that most of these cells have their own little engines and sometimes many of them!" Uncle was watching my expression of part amazement and part disbelief. "Just think: these trillions of little engines all need fuel! It is all part of their design – like an outboard motor, only more complicated. Perhaps these little cell engines work best on the right amount and type of fuel? What do you say to that idea?"

I sat silent: I was thinking of all those little engines. Uncle Wolfi, too, said nothing but picked up the oars and rowed on for a time. After many minutes he spoke as if to himself.

"All those drugs and all that surgery, necessary sometimes, yet it seldom gets to the root of the problem! But, you see, I had this grand idea – a brain-wave perhaps – that if I improved the overall food supply of my patients, this would give them a better internal mix of fuel as well as giving them better raw materials for their bodies to work with and then their bodies might work more efficiently; following from that, their bodies might start healing themselves and my patients would start to get better, only occasionally needing drugs or surgery. And indeed – Gott sei Dank – this is what usually happened!"

When Uncle started speaking about his medical work, his face changed: it lost that special smile of his, half teasing, half slightly mocking as though he could see a joke that others couldn't. He almost became a different person, all seriousness and concern. He was like that now and his look was searching, yet kindly. I was in awe of him at these times.

"Ah, little one," he said, bringing himself quickly back to the present moment. I was examining my hands in some puzzlement.

"But Uncle Wolfi, I can't see or feel any engines!"

"No, you won't," said Uncle laughing. "They are minuscule, but they are there all the same, right inside you."

"But not real engines!"

"In essence, yes. They are little motors, miniature powerhouses, if you like."

"But what are they all for?" I asked, intrigued.

"Simply to convert fuel to provide the energy we need for what goes on inside of us and, naturally, for our daily lives in general. Raising your arm to comb your hair or brush your teeth needs energy, you know," he added, "or staying warm or digesting a meal; even thinking takes energy." I thought about that one.

"Take movement," he went on. "Everything that moves needs fuel converted to energy to enable motion: if I row, it is my energy that is used, if I sit still in a motorboat, we fetch in the fuel for it from outside. Obviously, birds and dragonflies cannot go to a garage for their fuel so they have to make it from the food they eat. It works very well for them, it seems," concluded Uncle. Right on cue, back came our dragonfly, darting past us, chasing something only it could see.

I began to understand Uncle's drift.

"Uncle Wolfi, I know you are right about food as fuel which we then convert into energy, because if I eat sweeties, I keep jumping up and down!"

"Hmm!" said Uncle with a sigh, "Very probably! Yes, we eat to supply us with fuel and we also eat to supply us with what we need to repair and maintain of our bodies and, of course, you young ones need materials with which to grow big and strong."

"I eat because it's yummy and because my tummy rumbles if I don't." Then, having been reminded of food and giving a little anticipatory bounce, I added: "Oh, is it biscuit time?"

"Sit still or you'll rock the boat," snapped Uncle. "Anyway, it's time we were heading for the shore." Uncle's face had become grave, so I changed tack.

"Seriously, Uncle, you say that the dragonflies have their own food on which they keep well."

"That dragonflies eat mosquitoes and wasps, you mean? Yes, it would certainly seem that each type of living thing is endowed with the wherewithal – and this includes the know-how – to survive and thrive and multiply in the right surroundings and given the right circumstances. Part of the wherewithal is the type of digestive system needed to deal effectively with its food, as well as the skill in catching it!" His hand imitated the darting down of the dragonfly swiftly seizing its prey. "The know-how is partly inborn, partly learnt," he continued. "If, say, a butterfly's young can only thrive on a particular type of plant – and sometimes the right surroundings are very precise – then the butterfly will take care to lay her eggs on that particular type of plant, so that the caterpillar not only has the food it needs but, when it eventually becomes a butterfly itself, it knows where to lay its own eggs: perhaps home is the leaf of a stinging nettle," he mused. "Now as for dragonflies . . ."

But I was getting impatient and broke in: "I've got it! You put your patients on their very own dragonfly diet and, and," I went on, trying to contain my excitement. "And, hey presto, they get well!"

"That is not how I would put it, child," he remarked dryly.

Uncle always called me child when he wanted to rebuke me. "And I do <u>not</u> believe in magic. Hey presto, indeed! As if I snapped my fingers and people got well: getting well can take a great deal longer than that!"

"But what I mean, Uncle, is that just because we are human doesn't mean there isn't food that is right for us, that will keep our little engines ticking over contentedly and provide the right raw materials for us to repair ourselves and so to get well. Is that it? And will help me grow big and strong," I added as an afterthought to show I really had been listening. A smile came over Uncle's face, as he helped me out of the boat and tied it to its mooring.

"I think you are beginning to get an inkling of my secret. Well done!" he said, as we walked back to the house.

"But what? But which?" I burst out.

"And I think," continued Uncle Wolfi, unperturbed by my wild enthusiasm, "that you are starting out on a long and hopefully fascinating journey of discovery. May I accompany you? It would give me great pleasure." I nodded, speechless with joy. "I can see we need a little history lesson to get a perspective on all this, and perhaps a little biology, too."

We reached the doorstep of the house. Uncle had a meeting to go to and I would be leaving for England before he returned.

"So, Aufwiedersehen my little Fräulein!" he said, turning to me. "Till we meet again!" To my surprise, Uncle Wolfi held out his right hand and we shook hands. It made me feel very grown-up.

OLD BONES

I did a lot of thinking that year. When at last the next summer holidays came round, I soon sought out Uncle in the lounge. Uncle Wolfi had been listening to opera on his record-player and was in mellow mood. He looked up at my eager face and said: "Get your shoes on, Sparrow, and wait for me in the porch! It's time for my walk." We were soon outside and together we looked up at the mountains. "Imagine that all these slopes were once covered with forest. How magnificent it must have been! But it got too cold even for trees," he said, shaking his head. "And it was a long, long time ago."

I was bursting with questions, but Uncle insisted that we first walked down to the edge of the lake. We found a nice open spot on the bank amidst lovely alpine flowers. From here we could see the grassy slopes on the side of one of the mountains where lambs played together whilst their mothers ate steadily, seeming to take no notice of the games their young ones were playing. Nearby I could see the brilliant colours of a male pheasant, pecking for grubs; on the far side of the lake, cattle were lowing and clanking their bells.

At length, Uncle Wolfi spoke: "I seem to remember you

were suggesting that, perhaps, just as the bird and the dragonfly have their own foods, we too have our own way of eating, which suits the way our bodies work?"

"Oh yes, but I can't think what they would be." I said, picturing to myself one of the jam-packed shelves in our local supermarket back home. "There is so much to choose from. And I know my Mum says the ads on TV try and trick us into believing nonsense. It's easier for dragonflies!" I reflected, pouting slightly.

"Well, let's try and make it easier for ourselves. Let's play a little game." That sounded more like it. I was full of curiosity and ready for off.

"Shall we begin?" asked Uncle, making himself comfortable on the grass. "Let us go back in time about 40,000 years – by then we had long since developed into proper human beings. We have just arrived in this part of the world and are living as nomads at the edge of great ice sheets. We are intelligent, tall, strong and healthy." Uncle spread out his arm to encompass the surrounding landscape. "What shall we have for lunch, niece of mine?"

"Oh Uncle, you are joking!"

"Of course, but indulge me in my little joke."

"OK," I said, "I'll try!" I looked around with fresh eyes. It was actually quite bleak once you got away from Uncle's garden. Just rough grass, moss and rocks. No fields of cauliflowers, no greenhouses or polytunnels, not even an orchard except in Uncle's garden.

"It must have looked a bit like this in those days, don't you think, Sparrow? Colder perhaps, but the same sort of bare mountainsides: maybe a few goats rather than sheep, but essentially the same. There was a good few years to go before this whole area was covered in ice, sometimes miles deep. So, lunch?" asked Uncle, raising one eyebrow.

I was ready for him. "What about roast lamb?" I said, glancing up at the sheep on the mountainside. Then, as an afterthought, I added: "Preferably with chips and mint sauce. Did our early relatives eat potatoes?" I wondered.

"Much too early for potatoes," replied Uncle Wolfi, "but we might be lucky with a little mint. I know there is some water mint further along the lake. And it might have to be roast venison: it depends what we can find – and what we can catch!" I hadn't thought about that aspect of lunch, but it sounded all right. Thinking of food, I reached into my pocket for some sweets, but Uncle stayed my hand.

"Oh, no, no food until we have caught that deer. And that might take a few days! I daresay the wild ancestors of those sheep would be tricky to catch, too. Very fleet of foot!" Now that sounded terrible.

"But Uncle I would get quite faint if I had to wait so long for food."

"Not if you'd had a good hunk of game inside you recently." I thought he wasn't serious, but he seemed to be. "You see, we are organised so that our energy is constant, even if our food supply is intermittent," he explained. "If people felt faint after just missing a couple of meals, how could they go on hunting? Or even sit patiently and alert by a seal hole for three days?"

"My energy doesn't even last from breakfast to lunchtime," I said mournfully.

"Perhaps you are running on reserve? Too many afters and not enough main course?" he suggested mildly.

I didn't fancy seal meat, but tried to be brave: "Perhaps we could have some fish instead?" I suggested hopefully.

"Fish is thought to have come into our diet by then," said Uncle, considering the idea, "so yes, you shall have fish. Good idea. There's plenty in the lake. Perhaps you would like to catch one while I light a fire?"

So, fish it would have to be, and maybe roast venison or the meat of an early type of sheep or goat for supper if we were lucky. I looked around for some vegetables to go with the fish. There was nothing obviously edible. I looked around for some fruit for dessert. Again there was nothing in sight.

"Not a lot of fruit and vegetables," I muttered.

"Not a lot of fruit and vegetables," echoed Uncle Wolfi.

"But you said we were intelligent, strong and healthy," I protested. "Could we really be intelligent, strong and healthy just on roast mutton and the odd mint leaf?"

"Indeed we could," said Uncle Wolfi, "and indeed we were, give or take a reindeer or two, or the odd woolly mammoth." And before I could say another word, he raised his eyebrows and again said: "Lunch?" This time, forgetting all about history, we both happily tucked into the spare ribs with barbecue sauce which Uncle had so thoughtfully brought with him in a lunch box.

"Seriously, though Uncle," I said as soon as we had finished, "you don't actually mean that we could be healthy just on meat?"

"Naturally, where we live and in the modern age it is not necessary to do so, but think of living up here in the old days. Take our ancestors . . . "

"Have our ancestors always lived in these mountains?" I

interrupted, imagining our family going back and back in time.

"Oh, it got far too cold for that at times. People living here then would have had to follow the animals south. Perhaps, as the weather got warmer again, they returned. I like to think so. The climate here has changed a lot over the millennia, and so have the types of plants and animals that have lived in these parts. Did you know that, during the hot spells, elephants used to live here? And cave lions and grizzly bears? But that was way before the time we are talking about" Here Uncle paused.

"But to answer your question, yes, groups of our most immediate predecessors – before we human beings, that is – roamed around in this area for thousands of years, maybe 200,000 years according to some old bones that were found, and they lived entirely on animal food, both the lean and the fat. It gave them all they needed: they let the grazing animals do the digesting of the moss, lichen and grass – the insides of these animals had special arrangements which enabled them to do this comfortably – and then ate the grazers. This suited the tummies of our ancestors very well! And have our tummies changed much since those days? I doubt it," he concluded.

I stretched out on the grass and chewed a grass stalk thoughtfully. I eyed the pheasant, which eyed me and seemed to be saying: "Your uncle is right, you know! Mother nature plans things very well! See what fine feathers I grow on a diet of grubs, shoots and insects!" I am sure it winked.

LONG, LONG AGO

The following Easter, I was back at Uncle Wolfi's. The mountains were white and glistening in the pale sunshine, as Uncle and I took a walk along the lake shore. Easter was late that year and the snow lower down the mountain slopes was already beginning to melt. I enjoyed the crackle underfoot of the icy particles that still lingered in the grass.

"Uncle," I exclaimed, jumping with delight in a slushy bit of snow, "what did you mean when you said that there is always a sense in which we come out of what has gone before?"

"Just that, biologically-speaking, what we were matters to what we are now," he replied as he walked on.

"But Uncle," I objected, running to catch up with him, "you said that I was never to forget I was a human and not a chimp."

"That is also true," he replied simply, "and that is because of the importance of all that happened in between."

"Oh Uncle, you do talk in riddles!" I wished the snow were crisper so I could make a snowball. But I pretended to throw one at him. He ducked, laughing, and held out a placating hand, which I took. "Uncle, you do make it hard for me to understand."

"Perhaps if I talk in riddles," he suggested soothingly, "I

do so for you, the listener, to tease out the meaning?" I was getting nowhere.

"Let me try you with something very straightforward. Take food: Uncle Wolfi, what do you think we should eat?"

"It is a very modern concept this business of what we should eat. For the greater part of our history, the question has been, not what we should eat, but what we could actually find to eat. Choice seldom came into it."

"But that apart, Uncle, what do you, yourself, recommend? And don't joke about woolly mammoths this time, please," I pleaded, "or rhino steaks! I'm serious." Uncle Wolfi did his best to look serious, too.

"Well, now, let me see. I would say that, not counting woolly mammoths or rhinos, the safest food is still any that has been around for at least 100,000 years. So what was available for us to eat? Let's say meat, by which I mean most sorts of animal food, including birds, and perhaps the occasional egg. Next in time comes fish and later on, say during the last 10,000 years or so, the food of the herders and domesticators: milk, butter, yoghurt and cheese. However, this period begins to present a few challenges: first cereal, which was also a new arrival, later on sugar and then the ready-prepared commercial foods of the last fifty to a hundred years!"

"Oh, Uncle, you do make it sound difficult," I said daunted.

"I was just putting things into a sort of general perspective, a rule of thumb to go by. Start with the bigger picture, the grand canvas," he added, smiling to himself.

At this point I skidded on an icy patch under the slush

and Uncle suggested we climb a bit higher to where the snow was still crisp and our footing would be more secure. We made our way cautiously up a little hillock.

"I can see that it makes sense for our food to come from our immediate surroundings – in those days, as you say, there was no option – and that it makes sense to move around looking for food – ditto," I conceded slowly. "I can see that if you lived where there was a lot of snow and ice, there probably wouldn't be much plant food."

Here I paused. The high mountains all around me were spectacular, so much whiteness yet with big splashes of greys and blues and purples. I could see the whole expanse of the lake and its shores. I saw nothing move, no obvious wildlife other than a solitary raptor circling far overhead and then hovering. What had it seen with its marvellous eyesight that I could not, I wondered: a mountain hare, perhaps, but no, it didn't swoop but flew on. Uncle, too, had been gazing up at it.

"Wonderful birds, aren't they!" he exclaimed.

"But Uncle Wolfi" I said, returning to the question I had in mind, "If we can buy any food we want at the supermarket, why does all this matter?" I felt it was a good point. "And from any part of the world," I added, feeling proud of my observation.

"As I said," replied Uncle calmly, "because of who or what we are."

"More riddles! Well, I have a thought: the lot before us – our 'immediate predecessors' I think you called them – may have roamed over half the globe, but they did die out, didn't they. In fact, the lot before them died out, too. Do you think it was because they ate so much meat?" I asked with seeming innocence, adding: "I mean, they must have been terribly ill, all that meat and no fruit and veg!" Uncle Wolfi laughed out loud and his eyes twinkled with merriment. He had a special way of laughing, did Uncle Wolfi.

"On the contrary," he said at length, "to survive extreme climatic conditions, they had to be very fit and well. No, the 'lot before us', as you so disrespectfully put it, were a sturdy lot and enough of them did survive and breed to be around on this earth for longer than we humans have been yet."

"But . . . " was all I could utter at the time.

"As to dying out, they probably vanished for several valid reasons. Firstly, living by hunting is a risky business: what if the bison or reindeer herd doesn't come by one year and they simply can't find food?" I thought of the bird of prey that didn't get its dinner just now. "Secondly, for many years – maybe 5,000 or so – both we and they were living in this area at the same time: perhaps we were not too friendly towards them? We don't know. It seems, though, that there was some intermarriage, in which case they didn't exactly vanish. Just look at any large crowd of people nowadays and you will see one or two people carrying reminders of them with their jutting eyebrows, the flattened top of the head, the short neck and head poked forwards. In fact, it is highly probable that I have some of their genes in me – and you, too, Sparrow!"

"Me?" I queried, a little worried. I looked up at Uncle who was tall, slim and upright. He wasn't that shape, but maybe I was? I put my hand on the crown of my head to check.

"But, you know, it is nothing to worry about, little one, rather something to be proud of. After all, they had very big brains!" said Uncle, smiling.

"Perhaps," said Uncle thoughtfully, "perhaps it was precisely the meat-eating of our predecessors that helped give rise to us, that is, helped make us into the modern humans we are? What do you think?" Was Uncle Wolfi teasing, I wondered? "What is certain is that without our ancestors, there would be no us!"

"I'm not sure I like that idea," I said.

"Let us look at this another way. Now, what if that one type of leaf our caterpillar could feed on was suddenly not available? We've agreed the butterfly would go further afield searching for it. But what if that type of leaf no longer existed?"

"It would be scuppered," I said, "like the pandas without their bamboo."

"Scuppered?" queried Uncle.

"Yes, had it, bingo!" I said in explanation.

"This modern language!" sighed Uncle. Modern? That's what my mother says, I thought, as Uncle Wolfi continued resolutely: "Well, our forerunners were luckier in that there were several types of food they could eat. But as the climate changed and they had to roam further and further afield, the landscape changed, too, and they became ever more and more reliant on animal food. For instance, they ate the reindeer, which ate the mosses and lichen." I thought of our game of the previous summer: the lack of plant food on the mountainside and our imaginary supper of roast mutton with wild mint.

"Yes, I suppose so, Uncle," I replied uncomfortably.

"And so it came about that, especially – but not only – in this part of the world, the balance tipped more and more in favour of eating animal food, sometimes exclusively."

"But it's disgusting, all this meat-eating," I broke out.

"Ah, there you have it. Instead of respecting our heritage, such a way of eating has become 'disgusting' and we think of our forerunners as savages who are best forgotten!"

"It's true," I agreed.

"Yes, Schatz, it's true." So now I was Uncle's Schatz, his treasure, his little darling, not only his Spatz, his little Sparrow!

"Let us walk on," said Uncle Wolfi and I was pleased, as he might then change the topic, but no such luck. "Yet early man was far closer to us in kind than the apes we see in zoos. It is pre-man and early man – not the apes – who, over millions of years, paved the way for us. During this time many small but significant changes happened to make the bodies of our forerunners suited to the new way of eating. Amongst other things, there were changes in their guts, changes in the way their insides could digest items of food, in their teeth, in their jawbones and in the shape of their skulls; importantly, their brains gradually grew bigger."

"You did say that there was always change along the way!" I nodded.

"This process proceeded very gradually. By two million years ago, tools were being used and . . ." Here Uncle interrupted himself to explain: "By that time, we are speaking of beings we broadly classify as 'man', yet who are still not quite 'Homo sapiens', the humans that we are today. We humans only came into existence, that is we became the modern type of people we are now, roughly 120,000-100,000 years ago."

"Why does all this matter?" continued Uncle Wolfi. "The changes I just mentioned meant that, over that long period of time, the bodies of our predecessors were slowly but enduringly adapting themselves to a food intake made up predominantly of animal food. Note that these physical changes and also this adaptation had already happened by the time we first became who we are now." Uncle paused to make sure I was following. "We tend to overlook this, Sparrow, yet perhaps – and this is a distinct possibility – the very fact that that we ourselves came into existence as a unique species already fully adapted to such a diet holds a missing clue to our own well-being nowadays? In fact, what if some of our current troubles . . .?"

"What if?" I queried, wondered what was coming.

"Just what if," replied Uncle Wolfi with his droll smile.

RASPBERRIES

During term-time, I thought a lot about what I had heard by the lake. I went over it again and again in my mind. I longed for the summer holidays to come round so we could continue our discussion. At last I was in Austria again. It was a hot afternoon and Uncle and I were picking raspberries together in his large garden.

"But people didn't just hunt, did they!" I said, all of a sudden. "So people must have been eating plants thousands of years ago? You see I've just done a project on hunter/ gatherers at school," I added in explanation.

"Yes, yes, of course. Some people will have lived entirely on animal food, others ate plant food now and then, whereas some had much more plant food in their diet: it depended on where and when they lived and on local conditions. There are still arguments going on about this at the moment. But the hunting part was important. For instance, didn't I read somewhere recently that the indigenous aborigines of Australia always chose animal food if they could get it? As I said, I think some people are ashamed of our real ancestry, yet no other animal bows its head in shame when it follows its natural path. Imagine an abject eagle! Nowadays, do you know, they even talk of cereals as the natural and original food of man – not surprisingly, they are finding it quite difficult to prove. And we must be wary of results that are trying to substantiate a belief system. Of course I understand modern sensibilities about such things . . . ." His voice tailed off and we continued picking raspberries in silence.

"Uncle," I said, calling him back to what I was trying to ask. "Gathering?"

"I am sorry, little Sparrow, it is such a big topic! Yes, gathering. Well, imagine you are a bushman trotting across a desert: you have failed to bag the giraffe that would have fed you and your family for a week, wouldn't you relish any edible roots you could grub up and cook? Of course you would: you are well exercised and you and your children are hungry, and those roots filled an aching void and carried you through to the next proper meal. That situation is very different from wanting a bread roll round your hamburger, chips with your fish or pasta with your pizza, when you have already eaten twice that day, not to mention biscuits in between."

This last suggestion did not go down well with me.

"But I only eat biscuits when I am hungry" I remonstrated.

"You, child, have never known real hunger," said Uncle, I thought a touch severely.

"Well, it sometimes feels like it!" I replied rather sulkily.

"Ah, yes, that can be a consequence of, shall we say, too much of a good thing," said Uncle Wolfi enigmatically. "But back to gathering. We already saw there wasn't much of a selection to be had round here. However, we don't all live in the mountains of Austria, so what about round where you live in the North of England? What grows wild and is really sweet, would you say?"

"Honey!" I exclaimed.

"Technically honey is animal food and a rare luxury at that," remarked Uncle. "In terms of wild fruits, I admit a very ripe blackberry has a touch of sweetness, but have you ever tasted a raw damson or a crab apple?" He had a point, had Uncle. Raw haws were floury but not sweet, neither were wild strawberries. And I had tried raw elderberries and, after eating a few, spat them out in disgust.

"Now think of the fruit and vegetables of today," he continued. "Wouldn't you say that the sort of plants that grow wild, which are more like those probably eaten by early nomadic humans, are very different from the ones you get from the supermarket or greengrocer? You see, over the years, and especially recently, man has deliberately bred out the bitterness in plants and changed fruit and vegetables to be ever sweeter – even Brussels sprouts and cabbages!"

"I read of 'even sweeter sweetcorn' on a packet recently," I said knowledgeably.

"Precisely!" said Uncle. "So one of the things to remember when you are putting your food together sensibly is just how different the fruit and vegetables of today are from the products of gathering in those olden days."

"They were not half so sweet" I agreed, "in fact not a quarter!" I reflected.

"And this is something these modern-day promoters of plant food eating would do well to remember," muttered Uncle to himself.

"Come on: let's take our own gathering in for tea," said Uncle brightening.

"What say you to a bowl of raspberries with a good helping

of whipped cream, topped with a few of those tiny almond macaroons your Aunt Helen bakes?"

"I say yummy, yummy, I'll have food in my tummy," I answered playfully.

"Perhaps you would like to bring in some fresh dandelions and some plantain leaves to add to the salad for old time's sake? I know there are some down by the orchard. Afterwards, we will continue our most interesting chat."

"Oh, yes, Uncle, there's lots I want to know," I replied quite genuinely. But I wasn't sure about the dandelions!

After tea, we went for a walk.

"Oh, what a pretty little plant!" I exclaimed, crouching down to examine a mound of star-shaped leaves with a silver lining and stroking the soft silvery hairs on the underside of the leaves.

"Silbermänteli," said Uncle.

"Silbermänteli," I repeated, "Little cloaks of silver. How lovely!"

"Lovely in a cup of tea, perhaps, though not in salad" said ever-practical Uncle. "Quite tough and hairy – that's part of the way such plants adapt themselves to the cold, and even so they go beneath the ground for the winter!"

I was thoughtful. "So we, as early humans, had animal food as the main part of our diet, with plant food when necessary and in season, and the plants were not very filling and not very sweet," I summed up as best I could.

"Very good so far," said Uncle. "Yes, that was our basic fare for something like a 100,000 years and is what our insides are organised to cope with – and efficiently too."

"A 100,000 years! Wow!" This was beginning to sink in.

"And then came . . .?" quizzed Uncle.

"Cereals?" I ventured. I pictured all those rows of colourful packets on the shelves of our local supermarket back home and even sighed a little at the recollection.

"Yes, and then bread."

"The staff of life," I responded, remembering the phrase from Sunday school.

"Early humans may have nibbled the odd grass seed . . ." responded Uncle in his turn. Stooping, he plucked a stalk of grass and eyed it quizzically.

"Like Jesus and his disciples," I nodded, "and their ears of corn."

We walked on for a few minutes and then Uncle Wolfi resumed: "Maybe ancient peoples ate some seeds now and then, it is true, but not masses of cereal products and certainly not out of a packet or made into bread! What you probably don't realise is that when we humans came onto the scene the world was just entering the last great Ice Age. The coldest part was about 50,000 years ago. It then got slightly milder and the ice sheets advanced; they were at their most extensive about 18,000 years ago."

"And were sometimes miles thick!" I remembered.

"It was only after the ice started receding that cereals entered the picture. This was towards the end of the last Ice Age some 10-12,000 years ago, when the climate was warming. You see, cereals changed and we found we could grow them. Since then, over the millenia man has gradually bred cereals into something very different from their original wild predecessors."

"I love cereals," I confessed. Uncle ignored me.

"But that part of our history is well known. What is

important is that this introduced a very different type of food into our diet. Just because we can eat both plants and animals doesn't necessarily mean we can eat indiscriminately each and every food we like. Nor does it mean we can eat them in any quantity, I am sure of that," said Uncle with conviction.

"But Uncle . . ." I said, trying in vain to interrupt.

"You see, our bigger brains could solve bigger problems but I'm afraid we also created quite a few. Perhaps domesticated man thinks himself to be a new species? It is possible. And by wrong thinking he justifies eating too much of the wrong type of food – food that then doesn't suit the workings of his body – and it makes him hungry for more of the same?"

"But, Uncle Wolfi, if you give a totally different type of food to a species unused to it – whose insides are expecting something else – what happens?"

"Trouble!" answered Uncle simply.

TROUBLE

"Uncle, can things go backward?" It was my first question the next summer, as I had been wondering about this for a while. "For instance, if we chose to eat really like apes do in the wild . . ."

"We would probably suffer a lot of gut ache!" rejoined Uncle Wolfi with a smile.

"Seriously though, Uncle, would our brains grow smaller again?"

"Fair question!" answered Uncle Wolfi laughing. "It's not absolutely impossible, though naturally it could take a good few million years!" I was beginning to feel offended at his laughter, when he paused and said: "Well, done! You really have been doing some thinking! It does raise the larger question as to how far our basic diet is an integral part of our humanity, of our uniqueness as human beings."

Here Uncle Wolfi drew a long breath. At the time, we were walking together in his large garden. Uncle stopped and held out his hands to help me up onto a large tree stump so that I had a better view of the lake. "What? Such cold hands you have, little one, and in summer, too. Are they always like that?" he queried.

I nodded: "And sometimes my feet are freezing!" I replied.

"Hmm!" was his only comment. "Na ja, jump down

and we'll walk round to the orchard and sit on the wall. There's so much to unravel, like when a kitten has been playing with the knitting wool!" I put my cold hand not in his hand but in his arm to show I was getting older: I was twelve and was now at secondary school. As we walked, I imagined this tall old man beside me was leading me into a giant maze – there had been so much talk and arguing at school about diet. Yet, walking with Uncle, I felt content and somehow trusting. Anyway, we wouldn't get lost: Uncle Wolfi was so tall he could probably see over the hedges!

"Where do I begin?" he asked.

"You could try with trouble," I suggested.

"Yes, trouble. Trouble comes, but not always immediately, sometimes not for a long time . . ." Here, Uncle sighed wistfully. "Our bodies are quite amazing and bend over backwards to do all they can to keep us well: make do, compensate for our errors, bring in a whole host of balancing and emergency measures and so on. However, there is a cost to all this and, sooner or later, the consequences of this indulgence, or maybe we should say the consequences of this misguided practice, catch up with us." Uncle was losing me fast and, noticing this, he changed his approach.

"Now, remember you told me of how your neighbour was feeding a blackbird raisins every day for weeks, how it was not long before that bird came tapping with its beak on the window for more and how your neighbour was delighted the blackbird had made such friends with her. Well, yes, she felt befriended by the bird but it was really coming for its regular fix. It is like, like . . ."

"Like me going to the sweet shop on the way from school?" I ventured.

"And for the same reasons," rejoined Uncle, nodding his head sagely. "Not good, not good! So much concentrated sweetness, unnatural for a blackbird, unbalances the bird's system. Did you notice anything else about the blackbird?"

"Well, I know there were three nests built that year rather than the usual one or two."

"Interesting," commented Uncle.

Here Uncle Wolfi got up from the hard stone wall for a stretch and we walked slowly through the old fruit trees.

"And it is not just sweetness that does it, you know." Then and somewhat unexpectedly, he added: "Take hens: I did an experiment once."

"Not a nasty animal experiment, Uncle?" I said, immediately on my guard.

"If you call 'nasty' giving my chickens something like their original diet, I plead guilty. Naturally, I couldn't give them the grubs and insects they might have had in a Borneo rainforest, but I gave them shrimps and other such delicacies."

"And what happened, Uncle?"

"In short, my birds were much healthier and had lovely plumage, whereas the others that were fed on their normal cereal feed – and which came running for more – got their normal troubles."

"Is that why you don't eat cornflakes for breakfast?"

"So that I grow shiny feathers, you mean?" said Uncle, stroking the thinning white hair on the top of his head. Uncle was exasperating at times.

"But guess what happened to the egg production of my superb birds," chuckled Uncle.

"They had lots and lots of beautiful eggs that were even bigger and there were more of them," I suggested.

"Quite the reverse: the eggs were smaller and there were hardly any of them – in no time, the hens laid just two lots a year, behaving like the wild birds they once were!"

"But I thought chickens just laid masses of eggs naturally and that's why people like keeping them," I said in surprise, for this was a lot to take in.

"No, chickens are ordinary birds that have been long domesticated by us: they only produce an abnormally large number of eggs if aided and abetted by us in the way we feed them," explained Uncle Wolfi. "A bit like your blackbird, maybe, only hens have had years of practice?"

"Are you saying that it is the cereal that makes chickens lay so many eggs and for months on end? But why? How can that be?"

"It seems that, given in quantity, cereal – or rather what cereal contains – somehow disturbs the bird's reproductive system." Now, that had never occurred to me: how could it?

"Oh heavens! I hope it doesn't do that to us!" I exclaimed, alarmed at my own thought.

"Now you really are beginning to put the right questions, my young chickaboo! And yes, there are unfortunately many ways in which this can disturb us, too, ways you will no doubt learn about as you get older."

Uncle Wolfi noticed my anxious face and softened slightly: "Don't be frightened, Sparrow. After all, when we removed the cereal from my birds' feed, their reproductive systems did normalise. It is just something worth thinking about.

Perhaps a food, which is useful as a reserve to fall back on in lean times, can become harmful when it becomes a staple food, especially an over-plentiful one. Rest assured, we do have a choice in the matter." Uncle Wolfi now sat down on a wooden bench, patted the place next to him and I sat too. "When you feed an animal – or a human for that matter – with a type of food that does not belong to its natural past, there are so many things that can, and do, go wrong, some of which you wouldn't ever think were food-related. I have found that disturbances express themselves in so many ways . . ."

"Oh Uncle Wolfi, must you?" I pleaded, but he carried on:

"If, like our forefathers, we are programmed for a frugal and sometimes intermittent food intake, with the occasional, hmm, binge?" he looked at me to check he had got the right modern word, "you can see that a constant 'too much' constitutes quite a problem of overload. And if, into the bargain, this constant 'too much' consists of an unexpected type of food, there you have it! In other words, nowadays, it's not just all feast and no famine, it is the wrong sort of feast to start with. Na ja!"

I was close to tears. It was all too much.

"But we don't want to talk about all this now, do we, Sparrow? Surely, the good thing to hold in our minds is that we <u>can</u> eat in a way that makes trouble less likely and, moreover, that brings all sorts of benefits in all sorts of unexpected ways," said Uncle, smiling reassuringly.

"And our little cell engines?" I asked, not quite reassured, and remembering our time together in the boat three summers before.

"As you can imagine, these function most effectively on their primary fuel and they 'burn' it cleanly. With other fuel, the little engines have to work twice as hard for the same output, and there can be waste that is not always easily got rid of and can clog things up. You see, some of this less welcome fuel gets processed not in the little engines but in the cell spaces and without oxygen. I should mention that all parts of the body don't use the same fuel, but these miniature powerhouses sort this all out among themselves very well, that is as long as the overall supply of food from outside is in more or less the right quantity and the right mix. There is a lot of leeway, but too much of the wrong thing and there does come a time . . ."

Poor Uncle Wolfi, he did keep veering back to the thought of ailments, but then he was a doctor and that had been the focus of his life's work. Once he got going, there was no stopping him: "There might come a time . . . well, I have this hunch that if the fuel mix sent to the cells to process is too unlike what our cells hope for to function normally . . . then there will be too much fermenting going on and not enough oxygen around and . . . it is just possible that at least some of our trillions of cells will think they are again living in primordial soup and act accordingly." What planet does Uncle live on! I looked at him now as uncomprehendingly as I had when he first mentioned this strange soup. "And then. . ." he finished, throwing up his hands in a bleak gesture of impending doom.

Suddenly his eyes twinkled: "Do you believe me when I tell you all these things, some of which I admit are very unusual?"

"I try to, Uncle Wolfi, that is I do when I think you're not joking!" I said timidly.

"Believe it or not, I am not asking you to accept what I say. Yes, there are some things for which we have to take the word of others, but we can still do our own thinking. Never forget that! You see, for things to be meaningful, you need to discover things for yourself."

"When I first started thinking about the way we eat," Uncle reflected, "I doubted it all myself! I very much needed to prove to myself that I was on the right lines, so I tried my ideas out on myself just to see. In fact, for four years I didn't have any cereal at all and not many sweet things either."

"Sounds awful," I said, imaging life without bread, jam or breakfast cereal.

"Actually, it wasn't so bad at all," said Uncle, reminiscing.

"What happened?" I asked curiously.

"Less aches and pains and a whole new lease of life."

"Really, Uncle?"

"Oh yes, but perhaps what I did in those first four years was a bit extreme, so I eased up a little after that. That was over forty years ago and for me it has been very liberating. It is not as though I can't eat and drink what I like: I can. It's just that I choose to be very modest in the portion sizes of certain foods. But come on, it is getting late. Let us go in for our supper. I think you will find that the real proof of the eating is in one of your Aunt Helen's scumptious, if somewhat tiny, puddings!"

"Scrumptious," I corrected, glad of the chance to do so, but looking forward to the pudding nonetheless.

THE BIGGER PICTURE

I was sitting on the doorstep with my head in my hands, deeply puzzled, when Uncle came by. He stopped and looked at me enquiringly.

"I have a problem, Uncle Wolfi," I admitted.

"Can I help, little one?"

"I have found what you say fascinating and honestly it makes a lot of sense, it's just that . . ." I faltered.

"Go on," said Uncle gently.

"Well, it's just that I'm worried by the fact that it is precisely those things which must have been central to our original diet as humans that our teachers say are bad for us. They are going to be given red traffic lights!" I blurted out.

It was Uncle Wolfi's turn to look puzzled.

Presently he said quietly: "In the prevailing climate of opinion, such a way of eating as I propose is only thought well of by those who practise it and so know its worth. It is a difficult one. I stuck my neck out and I know the cost," he remarked with a distant look in his eyes. "My colleagues – those sympathetic to my work, that is – handle the problem very delicately. They don't advertise the fact that they use my diet in their treatment of certain ailments, but practise its principles discreetly both on themselves and on a one-to-one basis with patients," he said, as if to himself.

He paused, correcting himself, "I know I should not call it 'my' diet, and you know that, too," he added, I thought almost humbly. "And people can be so impetuous – I tended to be so myself – and too much haste can bring problems. On-to-one is the safest way. Yes, best not to shout it from the rooftops, even though you might feel like doing so at times, best not even to argue about it. Store inwardly the question: how could foodstuffs that have been an integral part of our diet for over a 100,000 years suddenly become bad for us? Foodstuffs so fundamental that we, as humans, owe our very existence to them? The emphasis of our diet may have changed very recently – or rather the script may have changed – but has the construction and organisation of our bodies changed sufficiently in the meantime to make our long-term foods harmful? Surely not! Watch, listen, read round the subject, learn what you can, but above all, as I said, keep your own counsel and your ability to think for yourself."

"Thank you, Uncle, I'll remember your advice."

"It's all very simple really: things work better when we are what we are, and are not trying to be something else!" I grinned: that bit was a riddle no longer.

"As far as I can see, to be healthy," affirmed Uncle, "yes, I know pollution, insufficient exercise and other issues have to be dealt with, but in terms of nutrition there is one basic rule: namely, we have to learn to eat and drink in a way which, as far as possible, keeps the workings of our body comfortably within the normal boundaries of the body's internal operating system. Overload is anything that unduly disturbs this working balance – and my colleagues know well how one imbalance leads to another!" he said, falling back into his own thoughts.

Eating and drinking in a way that suits our operating system – such an old man using computer speak! I was impressed, but I was none the wiser. I had heard Uncle Wolfi say similar things a hundred times, yet I still could make neither head nor tail of it. All this talk of being 'designed' in a certain way meant nothing to me. Then I realised that, apart from the snippets I had learnt from Uncle, I hadn't the faintest idea about how my body worked or even how it was supposed to work when it functioned at its best. No wonder I couldn't understand what Uncle was really saying. I shook my head despondently.

"You can learn all about it when you are older, Sparrow," said Uncle Wolfi comfortingly, "and if some day you want to try out the way of eating I've been talking about, I'm happy to be your guide, as far as I am able."

That evening, I still felt a niggle in the back of my mind: what Uncle said was so, so different from what my teachers said, even now I was at senior school. It must have showed on my face during our evening meal, because Uncle raised one eyebrow in my direction and went on eating his roast pork. At the end of the first course, Uncle Wolfi wiped his mouth with his napkin, folded it carefully and then beckoned me with one finger to come with him. Feeling both uncomfortable and curious, I followed him into his study.

"Now stand right over here with me and look at the picture on the far wall. What do you see?" he asked.

"Flowers," I said, "I think they're blue irises."

"Now go up very closely to them and have another look," said Uncle.

"Great splodges of paint!" I said laughing, "and I thought Monet was a great artist!"

"Perhaps he still is," replied Uncle Wolfi with a twinkle.

Walking to the window, he turned a thoughtful look on me. "Perhaps our knowledge of history – and of nutrition – is a bit like a painting: not exactly great splodges of paint, as you so charmingly put it, but certainly a brushstroke here, a flick of paint there. The trouble is people argue with one blurred dash of colour against another, and especially when it comes to arguments about what to eat. I don't expect your teachers say the same as I do?" Had Uncle read my mind? "Take all those studies one keeps hearing about. Often they claim to prove something after trying a diet for only a fortnight, or else they begin from the wrong starting point. Best to deal with the conclusions of such studies by holding them all very lightly. And never just read the conclusions – they can be very misleading – always read the middle as well! "

"I'll try to, Uncle," I replied.

"Little Sparrow, we all have a tendency to draw conclusions from little splashes as though they were exact details and not just a tiny part of the picture. It can be very confusing, and I confess I am no exception. There is still a lot we don't know. As for my part, it is now up to others to fill in some of the finer details of my own larger canvas. One man can only do so much. My hope is that by standing far enough back, the real picture will come into focus." I liked that idea. "I am fairly sure I have got the broad outlines correct. Yes, I think my bigger picture will stand up to the test, and that scientific research will prove me right in time. Did you know that there is a long tradition of using art to illustrate science? The ancient Chinese were particularly good at it," he concluded with a smile.

I hugged him appreciatively, but Uncle Wolfi held me at arms length and looked me in the eyes: "My advice to you about what to eat is to stay very modest with your intake of recent foods – and you know by now what I mean by recent – and then your own body will soon be your guide. It will tell you when it is happy or when you are overstepping the mark." I looked up at him gratefully and he continued, with a reassuring smile: "Treasure what I have told you in your heart, keep it as an open secret to be shared only when you feel it might help someone to know it: that is until the time comes – well, who knows – maybe one day, when you are older, the time will come when you, little Sparrow, will tell my story." I looked surprised but Uncle Wolfi at last returned my hug. "Come on, let's go and finish our supper," he said, offering his arm and leading the way.

Next day, I was down by the pond inventing a game in which Uncle Wolfi was a wizened old wizard with a long flowing beard and healing people with his wand. Then I remembered his objection to magic and started adapting a poem I knew:

> You are old, Uncle Wolfi, the young girl said,
> And your hair has become very white,
> And yet you incessantly stand on your head –
> Do you think, at your age, it is right?

Uncle surprised me. "What am I standing on its head now, little one?" he asked, mishearing me.

"Oh, I have just been going over in my mind some of the discussions I have had with you, Uncle, over the years," I replied, which was true.

"Well, you might be interested to know that I'm working on a new theory: I have been studying the history of our relationship to salt from the very earliest days, that is from the time of the single-celled organism onwards. In fact, I've been inspired by coelacanths. No, there are none in this pond," he said, following the direction of my eyes, "they lived millions of years ago. But, Sparrow, don't worry your little head about the fanciful notions of an old man."

"Uncle, you are quite amazing!" I exclaimed delighted, for to me my white-haired Uncle was himself ancient by then.

"No, no, child," he said modestly, "I merely try to apply lessons from history that are there for all of us to learn."

"Oh, you are not <u>any</u> old man, Uncle Wolfi," I protested, "you are the very old man from the mountains of Austria who had a priceless secret because he was so old that he remembered things other people forgot!"

PART II

WHAT IF?

After that memorable scene by the pond, I only saw Uncle Wolfi twice. In my teens, I was ever busy with schooling and exams. Uncle, too, though in his eighties, was still busy with his medical work and those magical summer holidays spent with him at his home in Austria became a thing of the past. My recollections of those earlier times dwindled into a mixture of reality and fantasy, yet the conversations we had together remained vivid. After my last visit, Uncle Wolfi and Aunt Helen adopted a pattern of annual migration, spending their winters in England and their summers in Austria. The large house of my dreams was sold; that must have been a sad day, for I remember Uncle Wolfi telling me proudly how he had designed it himself. Pulled down by someone wishing to build a bigger one, not a trace of the house or garden remains.

However, Uncle Wolfi kept in touch with his 'little Sparrow' – for he still used this quaint endearment he had used for me as a child. I had been fascinated by what he had told me of his journey of discovery and it had set me off on my own journey. I studied a lot, reading anything I could find that seemed relevant. Uncle and I discussed, argued and at times almost fought over ideas. Bit by bit, with his help, I began piecing things together. During our phone calls and voluminous correspondence, I had many chances to ask Uncle Wolfi questions and over time he sent me copies of his various German books. And still I puzzled on.

I had great respect for Uncle as an inventor. He had told me of the engines he himself had designed and that he had patents of them pending. I liked to hear how, in his earlier life as a medical scientist, he had designed a prototype of the space suit. Uncle Wolfi liked to think that he had inherited an innovative streak from his great-grandfather, who had constructed a very successful automated mill, powered by the rushing waters of the river Ache as it tumbled its way through the Tyrol.

Uncle's father, too, a village doctor in Upper Austria, had had a practical streak. During the school holidays, 'young Wolfi' would sometimes accompany his father on his rounds to outlying farms; in wintertime they would go together on skis. On these visits, he witnessed how his father not only treated the various ailments of his patients but would willingly turn his hand to whatever was necessary. What it must have been like watching his dad extract teeth or minister to their sick cows!

When Uncle Wolfi became a physician himself, it was as a problem-solver that he turned his attention to the seemingly ever-increasing incidence of serious disease. The shortest letter that I ever received from Uncle Wolfi, in fact, contained just two words: 'What if?' It was a frequent phrase of his, but that letter was especially delightful because, to me, it summed him up. Yes, Uncle W was a 'what if' man: a practical, problem-solving man who asked what if things don't work quite like that, or what if we have got it wrong, or what if we try such and such a way instead and see if it works? Uncle seemed to apply this question to theories as well as to everyday medicine. He was not, though, a random trial and error man: rather he was thoughtful and always looking for the reasons why things happened as they did.

My own first memories were of Uncle Wolfi as an old man and, by then, Uncle had a few answers and very challenging ones they were, too. So perhaps it was inevitable that I, in my turn, was led to ask what if, and even to put to myself the most daunting question of all: what if Uncle Wolfi was right? Right in his view of evolutionary history, right about our ancient diet being mainly of animal food, right about being tuned to frugality and periods of want, right about the link between what we ate and the inner workings of our bodies, right about us not exactly being designed for stacks of cake and biscuits – oh, Heaven forbid!

BARBARIC YAWP

I was in my early teens when I began to explore Uncle's ideas for myself. First, I needed to find the 'time before bread' that Uncle Wolfi had talked about, so I started looking into our distant past. I got so excited about what I read that I rang Uncle Wolfi, who was in London at the time.

"Uncle, guess what? I've found tough and hairy hominids, ape-men and tree-men and other ever less hairy but not quite men. In fact, I've found a whole family tree of our early ancestors."

"No, Sparrow, it was not a family tree: it was a bush!" he remonstrated.

"I can't talk about a family bush!" I protested.

"There were a lot of different stems as well as branches," he countered.

"A bush-like family tree, then? But, oh, how long it took each group to change into something else!"

"Yes, Sparrow, a long slow journey to mankind over many millions of years." I could almost see Uncle Wolfi nodding into the phone.

"Yes," I agreed enthusiastically: "Then came Homo this and Homo that, Homos with all sorts of long names and, eventually, we became Homo sapiens."

I was learning Latin at school, so I knew by now that

Homo sapiens meant 'knowing man'. I felt this to be a bit arrogant on our part: after all, our predecessors had known fire for, some say, two million years before we came on the scene and who is to say they did not barbecue their steaks like we do now? Uncle had told me that the last lot had bigger brains than us; they also had tools and wore primitive clothing and could make shelters like our own early kin. Maybe these skills had passed from one developing group to another? In the books I consulted, it didn't say. Whatever the truth of the matter – and evidence only seemed to come from the odd pile of very old bones and occasionally a complete skeleton with a few fragments of animal remains from the same cave – it was widely held that our barbaric ancestors were a pretty carnivorous bunch.

From all accounts, we Homo sapiens were also a pretty carnivorous bunch! This I knew in theory, as Uncle was always going on about it. It was the level of agreement among the experts on the subject that really surprised me, not only as to the predominance of meat in our diet over that long period of time but also as to its excellence as a form of nutrition. Time and again I found mention of the superb physique, tall stature, strength and health of early Homo sapiens, which they had no hesitation in attributing to their 'excellent all-meat diet'. Yet, in the past, Mum had made me feel guilty if I relished a piece of pork scratching that was to be given only to the dog! Something did not add up.

"Uncle," I said to Uncle Wolfi on another occasion: "as far as I can see, the experts all seem to think that our ancient diet made people really fit and well. I wonder what those experts eat for their own dinner? Do they try to follow the example of our ancestors or do they eat pasta and pizza like the rest of us?"

Uncle Wolfi chuckled. "I very much doubt that they want to emulate those whom they feel to be savages! Though I think some of us still have some sort of primaeval yearning for at least some animal food in our diet."

"I myself like a good Bolognese but not without the spaghetti," I put in.

"And don't you think it is possible that our genes remember that distant past?" he continued. "I saw a lovely story in one of your English newspapers. It was reported that a lot of London business men stopped to buy pork pies after work, scoffing them on the way home to fill in advance the gap in the low fat, meatless meal they knew they would face that evening!" and, still chuckling, Uncle rang off.

My next port of call was Uncle Wolfi's hero: the explorer Vilhjalmur Stefansson, known familiarly as Stef. Uncle said this was the closest I would be able get to meeting our Ice-Age relatives, so I borrowed 'My Life with the Eskimo' from our local library and I trudged, slid and sledged with Stef across the Arctic. I met traditional Inuit families who had never previously met a white man – this was at the beginning of the 20th century – and, oh dear, they really did live off animal food and happily, too, it seems. Further confirmation of an unpalatable fact!

However, the Inuit seemed far from savage: polite, welcoming and considerate to visitors like Stef and his companion. It may have helped that Stef already spoke their language, but I began to feel a growing respect for these supposedly primitive people. They fed and clothed their children, were kind enough to take food to other families in the group who had a shortage, kept dogs, made sleds, made needles to sew their own clothes and made their own copper knives to prepare food. They knew how to ventilate their snow houses, which they heated with oil lamps, and enjoyed singing and dancing during the long dark winter days. It all sounded very civilised.

Just imagine sub-zero temperatures outside and a whole family living in one room – and a room with ice-lined walls of snow – yet being able not only to keep the place warm, but to cook and dry clothes and boots with just one lamp that used whale or seal oil. Amazing! Moreover, while the cooking was going on, the inside temperature apparently kept at between 70 – 80 degrees Fahrenheit (that's 21 – 26 degrees Celsius, i.e. warmer than the inside of my house in the North of England), and the igloo subsequently kept warm all night. Yes, and cook these people did: they tossed lean caribou meat into molten ice that had been brought to the boil, cooked it just enough to suit their taste and then ate the boiled meat together with cold uncooked fat.

For afters, they drank the cooking water. Perhaps they, too, liked a nice hot drink, a bit like us with our cups of tea? I tried to equate seal flipper for breakfast with the sausage and tomato I sometimes enjoyed, but my imagination failed me miserably. One surprise was that, if sufficient food was to hand, these Inuit families chose to eat three meals a day just like we do, only without the snacks. All in all, Stef found a very healthy and robust community, who had attained a level of self-sufficiency and mutual help of which we could only dream. Obviously, life was not all roses: not that there were any roses, but there were flowers on the tundra in summertime!

I talked to my classmates about all this and they said the Inuit were only healthy because they ate all their food raw, and ate mostly fish at that. I thought about what Stef had said to the contrary. Here, I only quote one of his visits, but Stefansson spent very many years in the Arctic. During his time there, he found that some Inuit ate fish, others ate meat such as musk ox or seal, whilst some ate both meat and fish, depending on availability. And yes, sometimes they would eat their fish or meat raw in an almost frozen state, but it seems they mostly cooked it.

My classmates also said the Inuit ate berries and that was how they got their vitamins and that without these they could not have lived. I thought how berries were only available very occasionally and just at the end of their short summer. I replied that maybe the gathering of the Inuit was almost entirely of the animal kind. This suggestion did not go down well. In fact, I was not at all believed and I began to understand why Uncle Wolfi had advised me to say little. So I just muttered inwardly: berries, my foot!

On one expedition, Stefansson instructed his men to 'go native'; some were reluctant at first but, eating just seal meat, none took more than one to two weeks to feel comfortable and well. On another trip, detailed in his book: The Friendly Arctic, he was joined by three men who had ignored his advice to include fresh meat in their daily fare and who had been secretly living off store groceries for the previous few months. They got ill and steadily worsened; it turned out they had contracted scurvy. All three were subsequently cured with fresh fat caribou meat, lightly boiled for breakfast and raw if they needed further meals during the day. In two to three days, their depression had lifted, in two weeks they could walk ten miles and in four were apparently restored to full health.

Was this scurvy business where my classmates got their idea that meat had to be raw, I wondered? Then I remembered that Uncle had said that established illnesses often required stronger measures than did keeping the healthy, healthy, but all this did get me thinking. Had I ever seen meat listed under vitamin C on any of those charts at school? I didn't think so, yet vitamin C was needed to cure scurvy. This had to mean that it was not just oranges that had vitamin C in them. I knew that sailors took sauerkraut on long sea voyages. And didn't Captain Cook take live animals such as sheep and hens along with him? Hold it lightly, Sparrow, hold it lightly! I must speak to Uncle Wolfi about all this.

When we did next speak on the phone, Uncle laughed: "Well you know, you are not alone: Stefansson himself was not believed!"

"Surely not!" I exclaimed, a little shocked.

"In fact, in the late 1920's, several doctors were so sceptical about white men being able to live on meat alone – the Inuit were different, they said – that an experiment was set up in a New York hospital. After an initial check-up, Stef was given lean meat only, and this despite his protest, for he had seen first-hand in the Arctic the devastation caused by lack of fat he called a rabbit diet . . ."

"Sorry?" I said, not following.

"Rabbits don't have much fat on them," explained Uncle

Wolfi, "and when the Inuit only had lean meat to eat they got terribly ill. Of course, they couldn't eat just fat either, but to be well needed some of each. Anyway, as I was saying, at first Stef was allowed only lean meat and in just two days it had made him unwell."

"Bunged him up?" I suggested.

"Not at all," replied Uncle.

"Gave him the trots?" I guessed.

"Correct, whereas his former companion of the Copper Eskimo days, who was put straight onto meat with the fat on, had no such trouble. Once fat was allowed, Stef was soon well again. Both of them then spent a whole year eating just fresh fat meat – not organic meat or wild game, just ordinary butcher's meat - and with a free choice as to the amount of fat and lean."

"A whole year! Wow!"

"Yes, a whole year. They were allowed to eat and cook their meat in any way they chose: grill, roast, braise or boil Inuit style; black coffee was also allowed. The men chose mostly to cook their meat: his companion liked it medium, whilst Stef preferred it well done."

I held my breath in suspense as Uncle paused. "And what happened?" I asked eagerly.

"The doctors, professors and nutritionists stood around and watched, expecting them both to drop dead at any moment. Well, they didn't exactly stand round: they measured every single thing they could measure and were unbelievably thorough with all their examinations."

"And, Uncle, and?"

"Result: not a single sign of scurvy and not a single raising or lowering of any indicator that pointed to worsening of health. Stef, who was well at the start, stayed well and his companion who, as an orange farmer in Florida, had had a few previous problems with his gut, became well."

What can one say? To think of two men living in a big city being healthy eating just ordinary fat meat and no other food! It had to mean that meat was a complete food that provided everything that was needed. And now the experts were confirming not just that our early relatives really did enjoy animal food as the main and sometimes sole item of their diet but were supremely healthy on it. So what Uncle Wolfi had told me was all too horribly true! It reminded me of a little passage out of the long poem: Song of Myself by Walt Whitman, the bit where:

> The spotted hawk swoops by . . .
> I too am not a bit tamed, I too am untranslatable,
> I sound my barbaric yawp over the roofs of the world.

Uncle Wolfi certainly had a 'barbaric yawp' which he sounded 'over the roofs of the world', writing as he did of our kinship with 'savages', who ate little else but the flesh and fat of animals. And this our rightful heritage? Ugh! How could you, Uncle? You said as much during my holidays in Austria, but I suppose I hoped you had been exaggerating! And how ironic that you, a sophisticated person with no coarseness, roughness or barbarism about you – and such a lover of good food, too – should see such a barbaric way of eating as the blueprint!

Why, oh, why did Uncle have to tell me such things? It is not as though he, himself, lived on just meat or got his patients to do so. Yet I could not see his advocating the equivalent of such fare as hypocritical, for I knew Uncle to be sincere. Maybe it was just the words he used that were so off-putting. Uncle Wolfi himself ate sparingly, I knew, but not at all offensively.

I also knew how little I understood of the science behind all that Uncle had told me. Still, give up at this point I could not, and go on with my strange journey I must.

THE OLD WAY

I had enjoyed my reading. Yet, try as I might, I could not square that old way of eating with what was recommended today. Nowadays, any quantity of meat, especially red meat, was frowned on and any amount of fat in our food was a no-no. Babies should be given full-fat milk and even two-year-olds could enjoy, say, butter. Then, for some reason that I couldn't fathom, the needs of young children were thought to change and, by five years old, they were being warned off butter at school. From toddlerhood for the rest of our lives, we were told to partake of little meat – eating it three times a day was to court disaster – and to have less and less animal fat.

On the other hand, there was my remarkable Uncle Wolfi, who said 'nonsense' to all this and who made no secret about enjoying his meat. Leaving the fat on made it tasty, he said, and he was known to complain if the fat had been cut off. For Uncle maintained that as long as we stuck to traditional fats, fat in itself was not at all harmful and warned that, if we didn't eat enough fat, there might actually be a shortage of certain vitamins. He said, too, that fat only became harmful if we overate in general, and especially if we overindulged in carbohydrate. It was all very confusing. What was I, a mere schoolgirl, to make of it all?

Uncle Wolfi had written a book about his life and work as a doctor, which had seen many editions. The book was called Leben ohne Brot, meaning 'life without bread', though Uncle didn't really mean no bread at all, not for everyone at least: by bread, he was referring to carbohydrates generally, i.e. the sugars and starches that occurred in the food we ate. And he didn't mean life without any sugars and starches either, but life with only few. Once when I objected, he just muttered something about poetic license.

Uncle had kindly given me the first edition of his book as a present. My everyday German wasn't bad and I could speak it fairly well, but quite a lot of the German medical terms in this book were beyond me as yet. However, I was able to decipher most of the introductory chapter and was pleased to see that it had photos of Vilhjalmur Stefansson and of an Eskimo and a drawing of one of our ape-like predecessors. It felt very familiar and, now that I had read Stef's account of his visits to the Inuit, I was able to picture in my mind a genuine 'life without bread'.

It wasn't long before I was on the phone to Uncle Wolfi.

"Na, und? What now, little Sparrow?" was his greeting. That sounds unkind but I knew him well enough to see the raised eyebrow and teasing smile that played around his lips when he answered my calls.

"In your book, Uncle, you say that the Inuit diet provided all the elements our ancestors needed for good healthy bodies. What did you mean exactly."

"Think about it, Sparrow. Because the ancient peoples used to eat mostly animal food, this meant their diet consisted of mainly protein, some fat and a tiny bit of carbohydrate and that, in my long considered opinion, is an ideal diet. Ideal, mind you, I do not say sustainable or suited to the modern world."

"I don't think I'm much the wiser," I replied.

"Well, in our ancient diet, everything needed was present. Of course, the ingredients of say, wild boar still needed transposing into the ingredients that formed human beings as a unique species, that is into our own sort of protein, fat and carbohydrate. Changing food into energy and body tissue involves a lot of complex chemical changes but I can't help feeling that, in those days, this conversion was still relatively unproblematic."

"You seem to be suggesting a connection between what our ancestors ate and what their bodies were made of? To be honest, Uncle, I had never really thought about what I was made of. Thank you!"

This sparked me off on a new line of enquiry. In biology lessons, I had learnt that protoplasm, the basic substance of which all living things are made, contains protein, fat and carbohydrate and this now began to have meaning. All living things must mean that it wasn't just animals, but that also all plants contained protein, fat and carbohydrate. Well, I knew lamb chops had protein and fat in them – you could almost taste that they did – and that nuts and seeds did, too. But who would have thought there was fat in grass!

In different types of food, these three nutrients were present in varying quantities and in varying degrees of availability and hence usefulness to us as foodstuffs. I had seen a dog eating grass and then being sick and I had the feeling the same would happen to me. So my body wouldn't get much carbohydrate, fat or protein from eating grass! I now realised why Uncle had said we should leave grass to the grazers and eat the grazers instead!

In Mum's bookshelf, I found some biology books that had belonged to my grandmother. It surprised me that our own bodies consisted predominantly of water! Apparently nearly three quarters of us was liquid and there was water in our cells and water between our cells. We were also made of minerals and of very small amounts of the vitamins we are always hearing about, plus even less of the trace elements. Apart from water, it seemed that our own bodies – just like the diet of our ancestral relatives – consisted mainly of protein, some fat and a tiny bit of carbohydrate. This felt significant, though I couldn't quite pinpoint its relevance.

I knew from school about the need for protein to build and repair our bodies, but what did we want fat for? I had been told often enough that fat is just what we don't want. Fat collects on tummies and we try our best to get rid of it and, just by looking round my classroom, I could see that it collects in other places, too. In the old book I was reading, fat was referred to as a normal, natural, even vital part of us. I learnt that our very brains were made mainly of fat and that fat was essential for constructing our nerves; fat protected our organs from rubbing against or banging into each other and insulated us from the cold. Not only that, but fat was necessary both to the forming of our trillions of little cells and to the work they did, and fat was even needed to build the body's messenger system. We couldn't do without it; we couldn't, in fact, live without it.

So it seemed that, inside our bodies, both protein and fat

of one sort or another were essential to our bodily construction. Yet, according to what I had seen on television, even some of this vital fat inside of us was a no-no. I started worrying about what would happen if we got rid of too much fat from our bodies. What would happen, for instance, to our cell walls if we ate foods specifically designed to 'lower the level' of those particular fats that our cell walls are partly made of and therefore absolutely need? And what about our brains: would they be affected and if so how? Sparrow, just don't ask. It doesn't bear thinking about.

I was chuntering on to myself in this vein, when Mum came in.

Overhearing me, she echoed: "Sparrow, just don't ask," laughing at how I talked to myself. "Stop worrying and leave all that to people like your Uncle Wolfi! For all we know, the body can make its own special fats to keep things right. Let us hope so! Personally, I don't buy that medicated margarine they advertise. I wouldn't have the stuff in the house! Now that I am starting to eat butter again, well, who ever heard of vegetable oils being popular in the Ice Age?" Anyone would think it was she and not Uncle who had written about life without bread. "In the meantime, your task is to try and understand for yourself something of what your Uncle is saying to you . . . well, and to the rest of us. He is a clever fellow, you know, and didn't earn his distinction in medical science for nothing." Good old Mum!

So I did my best to stop worrying and instead concentrated on how our bodies operated when they were functioning normally and healthily. That day on the lake, Uncle had made it clear that the reason for eating was not just to keep ourselves in good repair, but to provide us with the necessary fuel for our existence. My books at school mostly talked of energy and calories and seemed to try and avoid the very mention of the word fat. Yet, from Granny's old books, I learnt that not only was fat needed as a so-called structural material for some of our internal bits and pieces, but that it was also our most efficient fuel. What a surprise after all I had heard about filling up with carbohydrate before a race and taking Kendal mint-cake up mountains!

I read on with enthusiasm. It was agreed that energy was necessary for heating our bodies and all other bodily activities like running, eating, thinking, digestion, going to the loo and playing football. It now appeared that, as a fuel to provide this energy, fat was just over twice as efficient as carbohydrate or protein. Moreover, our little engines loved it best and, believe it or not, our body's muscles – and this included our hearts – preferred to run mostly on the energy from fat. What is more, using fat as its main fuel, the body operated happily and competently, even if its owner had not eaten for days.

Had not eaten for days! Now this interested me, as I – and most of my friends, for that matter – could scarcely get through from breakfast until lunch without feeling tired or hungry or both. School catered for this by allowing us to bring in snacks. Mum said that, when Granny was a girl, they all had a third of a pint of milk in the dining hall mid-morning and, if they had the pennies required, could buy an iced bun or a doughnut to go with it. Then it was only two hours to go until they were given a hot lunch of meat and veg, fish or cheese and potato pie, with a substantial pudding to come after. Some schools even had tuck shops.

Yet I read how the Masai could jog-trot all day in the heat of the African desert without carrying special top up drinks or chocolate bars. I thought of the Copper Eskimo in the Arctic and how they would actually chose to go without breakfast on the day of a big hunt so that there was no fluctuation in their energy level. The organisation of the insides of our Ice-Age brethren must have been such that they didn't flag prematurely if food was not to hand. The secret, I learnt, was that nature in her wisdom had made it possible for our forbears to carry their own fuel supplies with them wherever they went in the form of body fat, which could not only be easily stored but just as easily accessed when needed for energy. And as for storage of this fat – shush! – I read how the Kalahari bushmen grew big bottoms to carry their reserves in. These were also peoples who, in the twentieth century, were still living in a traditional manner.

But why wasn't it like that with us? Why were we so tied to mealtimes and snacks? In my class, there were girls with big bottoms who got just as hungry as I did. I knew tired adults with lots of 'stored fat', who didn't seem to be able to draw on it when they needed pepping up; in fact, they said they found it almost impossible to get the fat to budge at all. The papers were full of slimming diets and how bad it was to be obese. Yet these 'primitive' peoples, given luck with the hunt, tanked up with all they could eat to first satiate their appetites and then to save against a rainy day. It didn't seem to do them any harm, so why did it hurt us?

I picked up the telephone: "Oh Uncle, why, why, why?" I almost groaned.

"You again, Sparrow? What can I do for you? I've only a couple of minutes."

"Oh Uncle, why was it good for the bushmen to obviously carry fat on their behinds and not us? Why could the Copper Eskimo have a great feast of seal or whale meat, store fat but not get fat and not get in trouble with their health? Why is it different for us?"

"Perhaps," said Uncle Wolfi slowly, "life was a little different then?"

"Yes, yes, I know that there was a long period of time in which you needed to be healthy enough just to survive: a time when there were no hospitals or drugs, a time before bread, baked beans or potato crisps," I said impatiently. "Personally, I don't think nature foresaw the 21st century!"

"Perhaps, it was the coming of agriculture that nature did not foresee!" rejoined Uncle, laughing. "Or, just perhaps, it is not nature's job to foresee but rather to evolve, to move from what went before into what suited the new surroundings at the time? Maybe, the bodies of your primitive people were working as nature intended? Remember that the long period of time you speak of lasted over 100,000 years and it is a real possibility that the system on which the bodies of our immediate forbears operated – of Homo sapiens, that is – was in place for at least that long."

"And still is?" Fleeting memories of those special Austrian holidays of years ago passed across my mind. "Chickens?" I muttered.

"Genuine biological adaptation can be a very slow business. Personally, I don't think there has been time for our bodies to adapt sufficiently to the very changed conditions of today. For the moment, forget today and keep learning about the ground plan, as it were, that is how our bodies appear to work according to the needs of times gone by. Do excuse me: I must go, Sparrow. Duty calls!" so saying, Uncle Wolfi rang off.

I dutifully got back to my studies, taking protein and fat and a small amount of carbohydrate as the normal diet of human beings. Thinking it through, I could see that for a people who needed to obtain their energy predominantly from fat, it made sense that, in the main, fat from the food was taken up for use by the cells more quickly and by a different process than that of either protein or carbohydrate, which first had to be diverted via the liver. I say 'in the main' as I knew it to be possible, in theory, to take up a little sweetness directly from the mouth, but how much sweetness was there in the ancient diet?

Both protein and carbohydrate, though not as efficient, could also be used as fuel to make energy. Even for our seemingly carnivorous ancestors, some carbohydrate in the form of blood sugar was vital for the everyday running of their bodies, and especially of their brains. Yet, there was very little carbohydrate in the ancient diet, often just the tiny amount found in animal food, But that didn't matter as no great quantity of blood sugar was required and, in any case, the body itself could manufacture its own sugar as needed. This was easily done by converting to sugar some of the protein present in the ancient diet, as well as the protein left over from body waste such as dead cells etc. – a useful cleaning up and recycling device, I thought. I read that the body could even, if really necessary, change fat to sugar by diverting part of the energy-making process to this end. As to the use of fat, there were also mechanisms that could be activated to help, say, the brain. How beautifully thought-through it all was!

For emergencies, the body did keep a small amount of carbohydrate in the form of animal starch. This was stored in the liver and muscles for the purpose of creating blood sugar – starch being just a lot of sugar molecules stuck together. This was one of the built-in mechanisms for times of danger, for example when the muscles needed to use sugar rather than fat to give an extra burst of energy for that fast sprint away from a rhino or polar bear. It was also a valuable failsafe measure for when food was in short supply. This stored starch was not designed for everyday use, rather it was a measure that called on the body's reserves only in cases of real need. This was interesting, in itself.

In times of starvation, when no food was available and these stores of starch had been used up, the body then had to fall back on using its own protein and fat to cover its needs for energy, including its need for blood sugar. The fact that the body used its own actual tissues to create the energy even just to stay alive was, it seemed, why people who were starving became so thin and weak. Grim!

All in all, the bodies of our immediate forbears really did seem to be organised with the expectation of little carbohydrate being present in food. It fitted that there was a built-in arrangement to restrict the amount of sugar to be carried in the bloodstream whereas, in order to transport it round the body, there was a lot of latitude as to the amount of fat which the blood stream could carry safely at any one time. There was even a little reservoir to help digest extra fat, if needed. This suited the type and variable quantity of food our forbears could expect; it meant their system was geared to cope with the occasional big influx of fat along with protein, as well as with their more usual moderate or sparse intake, depending whether there was a feast of wild ox, a meagre ration of one ptarmigan per family or nothing at all until the next day.

Nothing at all until the next day! The idea that, in those days, a steady stream of energy independent of the last meal was normal had quite fired my imagination: it was so different from the way I conceived things to operate. The past notwithstanding, I genuinely thought that everyone ate in order to give them the energy for the next few hours. Well, less in my case but, if I flopped in the meantime, I simply ate a few biscuits and could then carry on with my homework, no probs. But those were nomadic times with no permanent dwellings, no shops, no fridges, no cupboards stacked with tins and packets, no cups of tea or coffee at the ready. How sensible it was that our forbears saved reserves internally that could be constantly and instantly called upon!

Nowadays, in thinking sugar to be a better internal fuel than fat for general purposes – or even just for muscles – have we got the wrong end of the stick? Or, I wonder, in thinking that we can put on a lot of body fat and then sit around in the hope that it will burn off again when we next go to the gym or for a long walk? Surely on our ancient diet, at a time when fat necessarily provided most of our fuel needs, fat inside the body was popped in and out of storage in the twinkling of an eye, with our little cell engines chugging away in microseconds?

I learnt there were all sorts of controls to oversee the

smooth working of the internal goings-on, with many messengers to ensure proper communication between the various parts of the body, all sorts of adjustments here and there as needed. And there was something about a balance, an equilibrium to be kept between the use of substance to produce energy and the use of energy to build substance. A suitable diet, it seemed, promoted co-operation between our various body systems and so ensured that this balance prevailed harmoniously.

In short, what I learnt from all my reading so far was that the body was kind and wonderfully built to be healthy and, come what may, to make the best of things. In those ancient times and on our ancient diet, as long as people had enough food to start with, this system would have operated well and the workings of the body would have run smoothly. I couldn't work out what was different these days in the way our bodies were supposed to work. I asked Uncle Wolfi.

"Perhaps there is no fundamental difference," he said, "but as to a harmonious balance prevailing, I feel there is one important proviso – that the diet doesn't exceed a certain level of carbohydrate."

"And if it does, Uncle, what then?"

HOPE

It was about this time that Uncle Wolfi paid of one his rare visits up North. Mother was out when he turned up on our doorstep with a big bunch of flowers in his arms.

"For Sparrow," he said, handing me the flowers with a slight bow, "for my budding little scholar!" I couldn't tell if he was joking, but then I never could. Here he was: the same Uncle Wolfi, still upright, slim and immaculately dressed, almost dapper, the same droll smile that I remembered so well.

I asked Uncle in and, taking his coat, offered him an armchair by the fire. It was wintertime and he stretched out his long legs gratefully.

"Coal?" he queried. I nodded and took a seat nearby.

"Perhaps I should call you Wolfgang, now that I'm getting older," I ventured. "I'm fifteen, now."

"Please don't: it would make me feel old too! And then I might start calling you my old pigeon!" I let that pass.

"So Uncle Wolfi it is, then. Well, I think that your idea that the food we eat should be suited to our inner workings is remarkably sensible." I had been thinking about this for hours before his visit. "As you know, I have been reading up about evolution and also about the design of our bodies."

"I'm going to enjoy this," he said softly.

"But what happens when we have 'too much of a good thing', as you put it? And recently you mentioned balance and an important proviso, what did you mean?"

"Ah!" exclaimed Uncle. "Perhaps you would first offer your remarkably sensible Uncle a cup of tea after all his travelling?"

"I'm sorry, Uncle, yes of course, it's just that . . ." I was saying as I disappeared into the kitchen.

When I came back, Uncle Wolfi smiled. "Thank you. Most welcome. And how's Mutti?" he asked, as I poured the tea. 'Mutti' was what we both called Mum when I was in Austria.

"Mum's fine," I said, adding confidentially, "guess what! I noticed that she had been peering into your book and soon afterwards I found that there was full-cream milk in the fridge. I didn't say anything, but a little later I heard her telling a neighbour how she had been low-fat for 17 years – something to do with a hospital advising it for something or other – and how she never had digestive troubles before that, but has had them on and off ever since. I pricked up my ears to hear her say that now she's cut down on bread a little and put butter back on the table, she's managing a lot better."

"It figures," said Uncle, nodding slowly.

"And she finished by saying 'the old boy certainly has something!'" I glanced at Uncle to see if he was offended, but his eyes were twinkling just as they used to. Anyway, old boy seemed somehow right because, although he really was quite old, there was still something boyish about the way he used to tease people and enjoy little jokes. In one of his many letters, he had told me how he sometimes liked to provoke his illustrious colleagues with some new theory of his. "And I gave up sugar in my tea for Lent!" I added proudly.

"Good lass, that's a start," he said approvingly and declining with a small gesture of his hand the plate of custard creams I was offering.

When he had finished his tea, he looked at me with an enquiring smile.

"Where shall we start?"

"What I really want to know, Uncle, is why cereals cause trouble," I said, eager to get going. "And what trouble they cause."

"Ah!" he said again. "In my opinion, it is not just cereal: it is an overload of carbohydrate from any source. Though, did you know that archaeologists can tell whether old skeletons date from the Ice Age or more recently by the condition of their teeth? It seems that when cereal entered our diet, so did tooth decay! Of course, generally speaking, it is difficult to know exactly which bit of our bodies is upset by which items of food. If I said, for instance, that such and such an ailment was caused by eating too much carbohydrate, it would be very difficult to prove. In our modern life, there are so many other factors involved that it is difficult to tease them apart."

"I can see that," I said.

"However, I decided that one way of identifying a root cause might be to keep modern life the same and reduce just the overload of sugars and starches to see what happens. That is the approach I took. Or was it a biology lesson you were looking for?" he asked, adjusting his legs a little.

"Both," I said hopefully.

When Uncle Wolfi spoke in English, which he did well, he spoke slowly and carefully. Unfortunately, I cannot replicate his lovely Austrian accent on paper, as I felt it to be very much part of him. It was good to be with him again and when Uncle now began to get restless, said he had been sitting for hours in the train and didn't I think it was time for his half hour's walk, it felt just like old times. So we got our coats on and walked together down to the beach.

"You call this a beach?" he asked, gazing at the long expanse of salt marsh and the distant sea. "I see you have a cave!" It was a sizeable cave in the low limestone cliff that rose near where we were standing. I had often played there in the past. "That cave you have takes me back to a turning point in my thinking. It was half a lifetime ago," he said, smiling at the recollection, "and I had driven to the South of France to try out my new sports car." I could see Uncle owning such a fast car when he was younger. "Seeing the prehistoric cave paintings at Lascaux and Trois Frères – amazingly vibrant paintings of game animals such as deer, wild horses and aurochs – is what woke me to the reality of our ancient diet and its dependence on animals. Yet we consign our magnificent ancestors to prehistory: don't you think it odd that history only starts when cereals entered the picture?" I was all ears.

"As you know, at the time I was not in the best of health!" he continued.

"I don't think you were, Uncle," I said, responding to his understatement. I knew for a fact that he had been quite a wreck: had dicky hips, splitting headaches and a narky temper and could scarcely do his work any longer. And here he was still working in his old age! "But do tell me more about when you tried your own diet on yourself."

"It was soon after going to the caves. I had been a lover of good rich fare – and you know yourself what lovely pastries we make in Austria. Then, from one day to the next, I cut right down on such delicacies and I noticed with interest that my headaches gradually subsided, my digestion improved, I was much calmer and I no longer caught colds easily. What is more, the trouble in my hip joints vanished like magic."

"I thought you didn't believe in magic, Uncle."

"Sparrow, you are getting too much for an old man! To please you, let me be more accurate. Over the following few months, it was the pain and stiffness in my hips that just melted away and that, as you can imagine, felt like magic! The actual bony changes are still there even today, yet once I was well established on the diet, they no longer stopped me doing a little skiing or playing tennis. I even started looking the sportsman but this, I'm fairly sure, came more from the diet than from my moderate level of physical activity."

I looked at Uncle admiringly. He was a tryer!

"The diet gave me many years of freedom, maybe twenty, maybe more, but eventually I did need one hip doing," he confessed. "Perhaps I brought it on myself by playing too much tennis? And these days, my other hip does occasionally remind me of its old trouble. But we don't want to talk about me, do we? Let's walk on a little."

We walked for a while over the springy grass, carefully weaving our way around the dips and pools. It was a lovely day; the sun was already low and the colours in the late afternoon sky were glorious.

"So, Uncle Wolfi, to get well, you think we should eat mainly meat like our prehistoric relatives?"

"Did I say so?" asked Uncle with some surprise.

"No, well, not exactly – and, in the past, I have seen you eat ice cream and even pudding!"

"Quite. You see, my tastes are quite modern. Wouldn't you say so, Sparrow?" I was not going let his joking distract me.

"Then, Uncle, your basic message is simply: GO EASY ON THE CARBOHYDRATES," I declaimed, jumping over a pool.

"Nothing is quite that simple, Sparrow," said Uncle Wolfi with mild reproof.

"But it is agreed we need protein and I know that you don't disapprove of people eating fat, especially traditional fats, do you Uncle? That is, as long as they keep their carbohydrate intake reasonable."

"True," he acknowledged, and we walked on.

I was the first to break the silence.

"I have been wondering about this business of reasonable. But what is a reasonable intake of carbohydrate, Uncle Wolfi?" I asked, full of curiosity.

"What I see as a reasonable level is something like the level in our ancient diet but a little more, say like the level they used in Vienna before the war to stabilise patients with blood sugar problems. Fat was certainly not denied to these patients or even restricted, as energy has to come from somewhere. Patients had a free choice as to the amount of both fat and protein. In the common type of this condition, the diet was very effective, as I saw for myself, and even prevented the highly distressing complications to the eyes and blood vessels and so on."

"Is it really true about preventing complications, Uncle?"

"Oh yes, prevented and often healed. Of course, patients had to be willing to co-operate and to stick to the diet in the long-term; most did and benefited accordingly. You see, in those days, we could not rely on drugs and there was no high-tech equipment, so we had to rely on practical measures such as diet, based on close observation over many years."

Here, remembering those early days Uncle Wolfi became thoughtful and then said: "At the time, I did not realise how fundamental such stability was to the progression or otherwise of many other medical conditions, nor did I realise how crucial it was for our health in general not to upset our internal regulatory mechanisms too often or too much!"

"Our internal what?" I queried.

"We'll come back to that presently. I was about to say that the carbohydrate level prescribed in those early days in Vienna was what I eventually came to adopt as my basic therapeutic level," he ended.

"Was your level so very low, Uncle?" I asked with some apprehension.

"This level of carbohydrate might have seemed a severe restriction to some people," he admitted, "but what you have to realise is that, as a doctor, I was dealing with patients many of whom were seriously ill. By the time people came to me, as a consultant in internal medicine, they were very often already considerably damaged by carbohydrate overload. I found that I needed to use such strict measures to get results. Perhaps it was that my therapeutic level kick-started the healing process and promoted a change to a more appropriate gear?" Uncle seemed to like analogies with engines and cars.

"But for others who weren't so ill to start with, even a slight reduction in carbohydrate could start turning them around," continued Uncle Wolfi after a pause.

"I noticed you weren't surprised that Mum was feeling better!" I commented.

"A case in point," he replied. "You see, it is the digestive tract that is in direct contact with food and so, if carbohydrates have offended, it is often the first part of the body to make its protest felt. Fortunately, if the case is not too serious, it is also the first to be pacified when the situation is reversed and carbohydrates are reduced. I have found that adding fat not only satiates but also calms the digestive tract."

We walked and talked and had become so engrossed that we did not notice time passing until I shivered a little.

"Come on, the sun is almost down and it's getting colder. Let's go back!" said Uncle Wolfi.

As we returned along the lane, Uncle Wolfi told me about the good things that happened when people went on his diet. He said that it was not just their medical condition that improved, but that many of his patients also found benefits seemingly unrelated to their known complaint: they slept better; caught fewer infections; had less need for the dentist and had warmer hands and feet. As he mentioned warm hands, Uncle Wolfi glanced at me enquiringly.

"I know, I know," I sighed. "Yes, they are still cold, but that is just the way I am."

"Na, ja," was Uncle's only comment. "But that wasn't all: many patients found they suffered from less bloating of their abdomens; their stomachs were happier; their skin was in better condition and corns disappeared. And patients tended to feel better in themselves generally and a better mental disposition was experienced. Last but not least, most people found that they needed to eat less in quantity and less often. I have verified all this during consultations," he concluded. "Patients gained hope from such benefits and I'm sure this encouraged them to persevere with the diet."

"To me, Uncle, these blessings seem very similar to many that you yourself experienced in your own life," I observed. "I am impressed."

At suppertime, we had local roast beef and Uncle found it very good and ate heartily, but he graciously declined the Yorkshire pudding, the roast and boiled potatoes and the sprouts.

Uncle Wolfi looked at the roast parsnips doubtfully: "Are they vegetables?" he asked. Mum assured him that they were. It turned out he had never seen a parsnip before, so I went and looked up parsnip in my German dictionary and got a word equivalent to a country bumpkin! How we laughed! Uncle did however accept a small portion of trifle for dessert. Our serious conversation, though, was over for the day and I had to await the morning for our next instalment.

CHANGE

Next morning at breakfast, Uncle looked well rested. Mum enquired what he would like for breakfast.

"Coffee would be fine, thank you. You see, I am not accustomed to eat much during the day, but I do enjoy a good evening meal."

"Are you sure you won't accept anything else?" asked Mum, feeling a bit inadequate as a hostess.

"I would accept a cup of cream to go with my black coffee. That would be very nice." In the event, he also ate a boiled egg with butter and we felt that at least he had something in his tummy for his long return trip to London via Cambridge, where he was to meet a colleague to discuss a research proposal.

"I think you have some questions for me before I leave, little Miss Why-Why?" he said, turning to me once he had finished: "So what is it to be this morning?"

"Carbohydrates again, please," I said without hesitation.

"Now, you have been learning about the Ice Age and I see that you have got the message very clearly that, in those days, there was little carbohydrate in our diet . . .?"

"Yes, and what I can't understand is, well, why everybody doesn't know your 'secret' about diet needing to suit the design of our bodies – it is so obvious!" Then I heard in my mind the distant yawp of the spotted hawk: that's one reason, I thought. I pictured the shelves and shelves of starchy and sweet food in our local shop and the temptations in the window of the local bakery, and thought of the more-ish nature of sweeties, cakes, toast, breakfast cereal and pasta: there's another reason.

"From the expression on your face, you are beginning to answer your own question!" said Uncle, who had been watching me intently.

"But I have a problem, Uncle Wolfi. There is little carbohydrate in the composition of our bodies – that seems agreed upon – and you hold that there was little carbohydrate in our original diet, which seems likely. You also talk about fat as the main and most efficient energy provider. Yet, according to our school textbooks, it is carbohydrate not fat that is our main source of energy. How can that be?"

There was a lull in our conversation. Uncle was slowly tapping the fingertips of one hand against the fingertips of the other, as though he was thinking.

"You, Sparrow, have put your finger on a source of serious misunderstanding. You see, over the years I have noticed a worrying tendency to reclassify according to what happens in everyday life and not according to our origins or our inherent design. Take the domestic cat, for example. There is no dispute that cats of all sizes are carnivorous by origin and design and still are so in the wild. But now that the much-loved domestic cat is willing to eat appropriately flavoured cat biscuits, even some vets are designating them as omnivores. This takes no account at all of the costs that this so-called omnivory, so foreign to the bodies of cats, exacts in terms of cats becoming ever more subject to our own modern diseases. Sooner or later, this mixed diet makes the cats ill . . ."

"And the vets rich?"

"Precisely! And perhaps the same process is happening as regards our main source of energy and, like with the domestic cats, it ignores the costs to our health."

"I don't quite get your drift, Uncle," I said after a while. I thought of the medicines my best friend's pussy-cat had to take. Then my thoughts went to my family and how ill my grandmother had been – the cost of omnivory? "Don't you think humans are omnivores, then, Uncle?"

"It's the 'omni' bit which I have trouble with," he growled, somewhat savagely.

"Omnis, all or every," I remarked, displaying my prowess at Latin.

"Your Latin is OK but how is your logic?" asked Uncle, still gruff. "Take this: because we actually do something, therefore it is normal; because it is normal, therefore it is natural; because it is natural, therefore we ought to do that thing. Who steps back and questions the logic?"

I had no answer to that: "I pass", I said.

"In my view," continued Uncle, "we may well be able to supplement our basic diet on occasion, or even on a regular basis, with food from the plant kingdom. But the classification 'omnivore' must not mislead us into believing that we humans can eat anything and everything with impunity, especially in any quantity. I, myself, am sure we can't." Uncle fell silent again, ruminating about something.

"Perhaps it is time for a little biology?" I suggested gently.

"A good idea. That might help you understand a little

more about sources of energy," said Uncle, brightening. We were still sitting at the breakfast table and we now both got up and moved into the living room.

"Na, und? Well?" I said teasingly to pre-empt him.

"Na, und" repeated Uncle Wolfi and, changing language mid-sentence, he continued: "I think we have established that the advent of cereals, a food item full of concentrated starch, introduced a gradually increasing amount of carbohydrate into our diet. Lately there has been a dramatic increase."

I was thoughtful: "But, Uncle, we do have the capacity to digest some starch."

"True, and both plant starch and animal starch."

"If we can digest it, why does the increase matter, Uncle?" I wondered.

"This is where the biology comes in. It matters because, as you probably know, when we eat carbohydrate, it reaches our bloodstream as sugar.

"Carbohydrate of any sort?"

"Virtually any, and whether it starts out as sugar or starch on the plate, it enters our bloodstream as sugar: blood sugar, glucose."

"And?" I asked, encouraging him to continue.

"And eating cereals or any other foods high in carbohydrate, say, sweet fruits, creates more sugar than our bloodstream was used to receiving on our ancient diet."

"Doughnuts?" I queried.

"Doughnuts, for instance," he confirmed and then stopped.

"Let me see," said Uncle slowly. "I know that you are already aware that the bloodstream can carry safely only a certain amount of sugar at any one time, so why don't you put your little enquiring mind to work. I'll ask you the questions!" I quaked a little but kept silent. "If your body had too much of something it didn't expect and didn't want, what would it do?" he asked.

"It would try to get rid of it, of course."

"Go on!"

"Well, I could be sick or," I suggested, thinking of Stefansson, "get the trots?"

"Yes, that would work to immediately empty your stomach or your bowels and you would be very aware of it! But if that something was in your bloodstream, which you cannot usually feel because it is right inside of you?"

It was my turn to say "Ah!" But then I thought of our kidneys: "I'd pee it out!"

"As an emergency reaction to such a surprise, that is exactly what a traditional Inuit would have done when encountering 'white man's food' for the first time. Not expecting a rise in blood sugar, the 'guards' were asleep, but in this unusual situation the kidneys, which are never off duty and which filter the bloodstream night and day, did the honours, as it were. Well done, Sparrow!"

"However," continued Uncle Wolfi, "after a couple of encounters with extra sugar in the bloodstream – say the person developed a taste for ship's biscuits – this would change. Potential food would otherwise be going to waste. You see, our original design was necessarily organised around the principle of conservation and recycling, so our body was programmed to cherish every morsel of nourishment that we ate."

"Yes, it would be," I agreed.

"From that point of view, wouldn't an unwanted but

regular addition to the bloodstream require a rethink? In that case, what would your body now do with the sugar it didn't want in its blood stream?"

I reflected for a moment: "It would think 'I don't want all this horrid extra stuff. It is OK in the right amount but there is just too much of it, so maybe I could make use of it in some way: change it, store it, anything but have it in my bloodstream!'" I said, mimicking the indignation my body would feel.

Uncle smiled: "And this is precisely what it did – and still does. To rid the bloodstream of any surplus sugar, over safe limits that is, the body puts the extra either to immediate use or it makes it into storable commodities for future use."

I felt quite pleased with myself and thought that this was the end of the lesson, but no, there was a 'but'.

"But," Uncle was saying, "there are one or two slight snags to overcome: namely, in a body that has little natural use for carbohydrate of any sort and cannot store sugar as such, how is it to achieve either use or storage, I wonder?"

"It could burn it as fuel?" I suggested.

"It could – and it does – but to do so on a regular basis or in any quantity is not without its problems. Any ideas as to where and in what form the body could store the excess?"

"I suppose the liver might be able to convert a little of the sugar in the blood stream to starch and add it to its existing stores? If pushed, maybe the muscles could accommodate a little more of this starch, too?"

"Good so far! Yes, some could be used as fuel straightaway and a little could be stored as starch. There is a third possibility – and here is the rub – for the body also has the capacity to convert sugar into fat."

Change

"You don't say, Uncle!" Now this was something. "I knew fat could be stored as fat, but you mean the body can also change sugar into fat? No, don't answer: let me guess! The body then uses this fat as fuel, which, on the whole, is the fuel it prefers to use in any case?"

"Ah, now that depends on the modesty of the eater in respect of carbohydrate, and we'll come to that. Certainly it can store this fat, if necessary in large quantities."

Uncle Wolfi was serious but I began to giggle. In fact, I was so amused that I didn't even hear what Uncle had just said: "You must admit that it is funny, though, Uncle! All this fuss about not eating fat! We are told to eat carbohydrate instead and what does the body do? It turns the carbohydrate into fat anyway. It's rich!" I said, erupting into laughter. "What's more, first of all it turns the carbohydrate into sugar and we are not supposed to eat too much of that either. It's quite wonderful!"

"I only wish more people could see the joke," said Uncle, without a smile.

"So we may as well have eaten fat in the first place," I concluded, still laughing. "I thought it funny enough when I found out that, although it's supposed to be risky to eat much animal protein and positively dangerous to eat much animal fat, it is precisely animal protein and fat that we – that is our bodies – are actually composed of!"

"Well, it wouldn't be you if you were made of plant fat and plant protein. Welcome to the animal kingdom, my little soya bean!" said Uncle wryly.

"But that we can turn the carbohydrate we eat into fat when it gets inside of us, and into animal fat at that, is the best yet," I said, wiping the tears of merriment from my eyes.

"I'm glad you see the irony," said Uncle Wolfi, standing up and walking round the room. "Clever isn't it, rendering an unwanted substance potentially useful!"

"Very green," I readily acknowledged, trying to pay attention once again.

"In both senses of the word!" said Uncle with a teasing smile. "It recycles, yes, but the measure is naïve – or should I say it does not readily work to our advantage – as neither the liver nor the muscles have any desire to store much extra starch. And even the fatty tissue can be stretched! That is a pun, you see. Well, the fat cells do in fact stretch to accommodate the extra fat to be stored and they also grow in number. All this is fair enough if these measures are required only occasionally . . ." Uncle broke off mid-sentence to ask: "Can you spot any possible problems, little Sparrow?"

"I have been wondering why very fat people aren't always bouncing with energy: they should be with all that stored fat at their disposal. Skinny rabbits like me have more zip! I can't make it out."

"Can you guess?"

"I'm still trying to get my head round it," I said quite honestly and, as he was still pacing round the living room, I added: "Uncle, I am wondering whether you would like a proper walk? Do you have time?"

"I don't have to leave for an hour or so. Yes, lets go."

THE PEPPERPOT

In no time, well wrapped up against the cold, Uncle Wolfi and I were off through the hazel copse at the end of our road and on towards the long ridge of mixed woodland. Here, a pair of peregrine falcons roosted; I had seen father and son carry off white doves from our neighbour's roof. I don't think I would have liked to be a real sparrow with those birds around! Soon we were in the wood, ambling together through paths deep with leaf mould. It smelt wonderful and Uncle looked happy.

"In those days, the guards were only called out when there was a real emergency!" he said, quite out of the blue. We had arrived at a clearing from where there was a pleasing view over the bay and surrounding area. "On their regular routine duty, they co-operated so harmoniously that people would have scarcely known of their existence. These days, it is so different. Enter carbohydrates and the guards have to scramble to their posts and are lucky if they have time off at all!" I looked at him enquiringly. "So much time spent dealing with the problem of sugar," he said in explanation.

We were standing above the surrounding trees, next to a dumpy but rather charming little monument locally called the pepperpot, and Uncle raised his eyes to survey the hazy blue hills in the distance. Nowadays . . ." here Uncle was shaking his head and gazing wistfully at the view, "nowadays we have to call far too often on our regulatory system to sort out the problems we ourselves have created."

For the moment, Uncle Wolfi seemed to have quite forgotten my existence so I walked several times round the pepperpot, glimpsing now the inland hills, now peering in vain into some nearby hazel bushes to see if the squirrels had left any nuts and now appreciating the wide expanse of the bay and the distant sea. Eventually, I touched Uncle on the elbow: "Uncle, our regulatory system?" This was something new and I was interested.

"Ah yes," he said, gathering his thoughts together. "You have to bear in mind that we evolved geared to frugality, but over the millennia, and especially recently, there has been a fundamental shift to abundance, even to overabundance: in other words, a shift from a sometimes 'too little' to an often 'too much'. I am speaking here of the Western world and particularly of carbohydrates. From this perspective, you can see the adjustments which the body has to make to this new situation puts great demands on those bits of us that try to keep our bodies running smoothly, and often overtaxes them considerably."

I waited eagerly.

"Let us sit down and I'll explain as best I can." We found a group of nearby rocks to sit on and Uncle continued: "We have agreed that unwanted sugar must be removed from the bloodstream and either put to use or stored. But who or what is to see to it? Who, let us say, is to give the orders in this new discordant situation?"

"Is this is where the guards come in?"

"It is and there is, in fact, a whole group of guards – or shall we call them controllers – working together inside of us. These controllers all have their routine duties to perform, as I said, but now there is an extra task of great urgency. Removing excess sugar is so crucial to our health that not only is the whole group of controllers mobilised in one way or another to achieve this but there needs to be a pecking order. Perhaps not surprisingly, the controller whose specific job it is to monitor the level of sugar in the bloodstream gains particular importance. Let us call him Controller No.1."

"He's the Fat Controller!" It was my turn to make a pun, but Uncle didn't get it.

"In more sense than one," he said seriously, "as you will see." One of the tasks of Controller No.1 is to organise the conversion of sugar to fat to put into storage, another is to tell the body cells to make energy by 'burning' sugar rather than fat or protein. Together with its associates, Controller No.2 has always had the job of mobilising fat for energy use, but this would now create a conflict of purpose, therefore No.1 tells No.2 that he must not do so, for the moment at any rate."

"And I bet the orders of No.1 must be obeyed!"

"Quite so," said Uncle.

We walked on in order to see if we could get a better glimpse of the shore line, but were soon back amongst the trees. I scuffled the leaves underfoot.

"So, it is Controller No.1 which has to make sure our cells with their little engines switch to using sugar instead," I reiterated to check I had understood.

Uncle nodded: "That's one job, certainly, but you've left

out another important one. Think about it: if the carbohydrate consumption continues to be immoderate, and especially if a sugary or starchy snack is also eaten between meals – as so often happens with morning tea or afternoon coffee breaks and even at bed-time, too – then?"

"Controller No.1 has to go on working overtime to see to this."

"Correct. And?"

"Oh, Uncle, I'm tired with so much thinking!" I complained. "It uses up so much energy," I added to show I had at least learnt something. Uncle gave me a moment to do a cartwheel among the leaves.

"I'll help you get your thinking cap back on. What is our biggest – and potentially huge – storage depot for all that unwanted extra sugar?"

"The fat tissues," I exclaimed, "and Fat Controller No.1 has a grand time ordering the extra sugar to be changed into fat and sent there."

"Good! Can you work out what happens then?"

"Well, if it's urgent to use up sugar, it's no good allowing fat to be used to make energy, so our bossy Fat Controller puts his foot down and doesn't allow any fat to be released from storage at all!" I said proudly.

"You have got it! Result: not only does the body have to run on sugar as its main fuel but little fat is released and ever more fat is stored. Go and do another bit of your fancy gymnastics as I have another question for you." I did as requested.

"Listen carefully, because this next bit is important. If the over consumption of carbohydrates continues over the years, can you imagine the result? Here you have to think of the cumulative effort of the situation. I'll give you a clue: too many sugars and starches eaten = too much fat created and stored by the body = ?"

"Very fat people!"

"Precisely: very fat people," confirmed Uncle Wolfi.

"Very fat people," I reiterated. "It seems too simple to be true."

"Yet, logically, the more carbohydrates eaten, the more sugar there is in the bloodstream to get rid of, and, if not immediately used for energy, the more fat is destined for the fat tissues," repeated Uncle in his turn. "Obesity can indeed be as simple as that."

"Don't people realise?" I exclaimed, scarcely believing what I was hearing.

"Lack of energy often accompanies obesity and there are other costs not so visible," continued Uncle Wolfi, ignoring my incredulity. "Of course, there can be many stages and many complications along the way, but in essence that is the process."

After a few minutes cogitation, a thought struck me: "Costs and complications? But I thought the controllers were supposed to be on our side and would try to do the best for us at all times," I said, protesting slightly.

"There is an answer to that, Sparrow. You see, there is short-term wisdom and long-term wisdom. The body has to react with short-term wisdom especially when safeguarding the sugar levels in the blood stream and cannot at the same time act in a way which might prevent problems later on." I could see that yes, the body was still on our side and I said as much.

"Remember that it is not fat per se that makes us fat – not the fat we eat, anyway," commented Uncle, "as it does not disturb our controllers in the same way. "Ironically, eating fat can help you, not put on, but lose body fat!" Uncle was losing me again. "In fact, I feel that the current level of obesity in our society is wholly preventable, but there is one important proviso. . ."

"One important proviso," I echoed. That rang a bell.

"That we don't eat too many carbohydrates!" we chorused in unison and we both laughed together.

"There is another scenario, which I have never fully understood," said Uncle Wolfi, growing serious again. "It is the other side of the coin, if you like: some people eat a lot of carbohydrate and get thinner, are more restless and are ever on the go."

"Perhaps too much sugar goes to their muscles and they have to burn it off in mega activity?"

"Yes, perhaps."

"Skinny people like me do seem to get faster and faster! Or could there be other controllers who get huffy or bossy, or just speed things up?"

"Yes, perhaps that, too, if I understand you correctly."

"But the picture is not all doom and gloom", added Uncle Wolfi reassuringly. "If consumption of carbohydrate is not too high – and for many people who eat modestly this is still the case – then Controller No.1 rules the roost for a couple of hours or so after a meal, but after that he steps down allowing Controller No.2 to order fat to be used for fuel once more. This includes the fat made from the carbohydrate we eat!"

"A sort of working compromise between then and now?" I put in.

"Yes, if you like. In fact, this pattern is seen so frequently that is now described as normal. For some people, this arrangement can go on for many years fairly unproblematically, occasionally lifelong, and as a result reasonable health and normal weight can be maintained, especially in those that are active, have a sound constitution, good heredity and, as I said, who don't overeat generally."

"A tall order!" I mused, "but good news for some."

"Good news for some, certainly. However, take heredity. If you come from generations of overeaters of carbohydrate or even just have, say, overweight parents, things often don't run as smoothly as they might otherwise. Even so problems are not inevitable if remedial action is taken. I have noticed that trouble seems to get earlier by the generation, and especially since this craze for reducing even traditional fats." Uncle sighed. I sighed, too, at that ominous word 'trouble'.

"Does this answer your question about our main source of energy, Sparrow?" I hesitated. "It is all too easy to confuse carbohydrates on the plate with carbohydrates as they are used by the body internally because, once eaten, carbohydrates may still exist as sugar or starch or they may have been changed into fat. So we have to be quite clear what we are talking about."

"Very clear," I agreed.

"Let me recap," suggested Uncle. "Now, in your country and mine, there is plenty of choice as to what we can eat. For those who choose to eat little carbohydrate, the main dietary source of energy is likely to be fat. I know it is for me. And therefore the main internal source of energy is also likely to be fat."

"In our little cell engines?"

"Yes, Sparrow, in the little cell engines. When people eat slightly more carbohydrate, this amount of carbohydrate may or may not form the main dietary source of energy. The bodies of these people run, not exactly on half and half, but their cells alternate between using mainly carbohydrate and using mainly fat to make energy, and do so fairly comfortably, as you know."

"The working compromise?"

"Quite so. Once the consumption of carbohydrate becomes, shall we say, immoderate, then carbohydrate becomes not only our main dietary source of energy but also our main source of energy at cell level. This is because, as already explained, to save our very lives the 'burning' of excess sugar as fuel has to take priority over the use of fat – the body has no choice in the matter."

"So you see," concluded Uncle, "the fact of the matter is simply that the more carbohydrate we eat, and I am talking of quantity not of percentages, the more that carbohydrate actually does become our main source of energy, whether as regards the menu or as regards our insides."

"Oh Uncle," I said, and fell silent. I knew he was right.

"This new reality is rapidly becoming the norm in everyday life. Confusion results and the thin line between truth and error is crossed. The link with our past is broken; any idea as to what ought to be our main internal energy source according to our origin as a species or according to the inherent design of our bodies – and so any notion as to best practice – is lost. It may be true that for many people carbohydrate has become their main internal source of energy, but this by no means implies that carbohydrate is therefore the natural, most efficient and most health-promoting main source of fuel for us. That it is the most desirable source of energy at cell level is very definitely an error, an error too often leading to widespread and disastrous consequences for our health and well-being. And there you have it!"

Here Uncle looked at his watch and then at me. "But worry not, niece of mine," he said gently. "Just always remember that we do have a choice in the matter."

"Sparrow, now that you are beginning to 'get my drift', as you put it," Uncle said, as we walked homewards, "would you consider being useful to me? Writing English I find so much more difficult than speaking it and I want to write an article or two about my work while I'm in London. I am also thinking of working on a summary of Leben ohne Brot in English. Of course, I'll do all the notes and technical terms – and there won't be words like 'narky', 'scuppered' or 'probs'. If I make notes, would you write it out in good English? I know you are capable. I would be so pleased if you would."

"I'll try, Uncle Wolfi, I'll try," I said, honoured as well as overawed by the request.

When we got back to the house, there was only time for a hot drink. Soon the taxi came. We all said our farewells and Uncle was off and away.

PART III

HOMEWORK

To be worthy of Uncle Wolfi's trust, I had plenty of homework to do. The week after his visit, Uncle sent me a copy of what he called his 'red book'. Over the years, Uncle had added lots of extra bits to his main book, Leben ohne Brot, and it had run into many editions – nine, I think – before being translated. But here it was in English, Dismantling a Myth: the Role of Fat and Carbohydrates in our Diet, my very own red book.

Full of curiosity, I started reading. In it, Uncle began by saying that there had been doctors before him who had had similar ideas about diet. Even at the time of his 'awakening' some fifty years ago, there was a doctor, very high up in the medical profession in America, who was putting his patients on a diet more extreme than Uncle's. Meat, meat fat and coffee, I think I read, which seemed very much like what Stef ate during his experimental year in New York, except that this doctor permitted the occasional vegetable. Uncle, I knew, was far more liberal than that, for I hadn't forgotten those delicious puddings I had eaten at his home in Austria as a child.

In his book, Uncle Wolfi tells the story of how, through his work as a doctor, he came to connect the eating of carbohydrates, especially too many carbohydrates, with various bodily upsets. It was quite early on in his work as a doctor that Uncle had grown fascinated by problems to do with the internal regulation of our bodies and in particular the interplay between different disturbances. In a preface, it said that he was one of the first to spot certain links in this area. For my sake, Uncle had called these upsettable regulators 'controllers', a term I continued to use, as it is how thing operate that most interested me.

Uncle Wolfi did make an attempt to make this book intelligible to people like me who weren't medics. I liked, for example, the way Uncle talked about the 'sugar squad' when referring to the group of controllers responsible for keeping the level of blood sugar within safe bounds. I liked, too, the way he described living on our present mixed diet as rather like the experience of driving a sports car on inferior, and not quite suitable, regular petrol, as compared with the delightfully smooth run driving such a car on super. Not that I had ever even ridden in a sports car, but this appealed to my imagination.

However, he also wrote with his fellow doctors in mind and I confess the book was generally hard going for me. I was dazzled by the complicated names and technical phrases, and then there were so many diseases. Perhaps I was not yet old enough to cope with thinking about all those bits of people that can go wrong. I therefore contented myself with trying to understand a bit more about the basic processes that Uncle had started explaining to me.

I learnt that our body works as a whole and that our health depends on every part of the body co-operating in a co-ordinated effort. I learnt, too, that the special controllers, which Uncle took such an interest in, had their seats in the various glands, each having its own task or tasks to perform yet all needing to pull together. They worked under a big boss, situated in the brain, and all of them sent their instructions for various bodily processes straight into the blood stream but, as Uncle had explained, Controller No.1 could weigh in and give orders to the others in the squad in the event of a blood sugar emergency.

I still thought the body was kind and doing its best for us in all situations and yes, the controllers shared and adjusted to each other's workloads. I could see that if one controller was called on to do more than usual, then another might have to do less to make this possible, and how sometimes there needed to be a particular type of teamwork for them to achieve the same goal. I could also see that if you upset one controller too much, then this might upset the others in a sort of chain reaction. And it wasn't just the controllers, there were layer upon layer of related activities going on inside us which were also affected, and this chain could go on and on until there was disturbance so far removed from the beginning of the chain that its origin was lost to view. Phew!

It all made a sort of sense to me, but it didn't make it any clearer why someone's corns disappeared if they ate fewer carbohydrates! I suppose one answer was that, as Uncle had said, skin quality improved. But then what had skin quality to do with eating sugars and starches? Ah – a glimmer of light! One possible answer was that eating less carbohydrate imposed less restriction on the controller in charge of skin quality. Could this be our Controller No.2? For Uncle seemed to think that when told to go easy on fat being fetched from the fat cells, this affected No.2's ability to perform other duties, such as seeing to the fighting of infection and to supervising growth and repair. Would neglected skin renewal and repair make one more liable to corns? It had to be possible and Uncle had said his skin became more resilient and chafed less. This was getting exciting.

In the wake of this thought, I began to see why, with the intake of carbohydrate much reduced, there was a chance for real collaboration between the controllers to keep our body strong and healthy. Controller No.2, his work no longer hampered by Controller No.1, could now see to the ongoing work of renewal and repair and with No.1 no longer forcing the cells to use sugar for making energy, No.2 could instruct the release of any necessary fat and the cells were again free to choose the fuel to suit the purpose in hand, whether fat, protein or carbohydrate. In effect, by restricting carbohydrate, the key was restored to the previously locked food cupboard. Was this the sort of thing hinted at by Uncle's comment about harmony prevailing only if . . .? Co-operation was certainly more constructive than opposition.

However, it turned out that unlocking the food cupboard was not always so simple and that changes consequent on eating carbohydrate were not always easy to reverse. Overeating carbohydrates might cause a great accumulation of body fat, for instance, but this in itself led to alterations in the balance of controller activity. Uncle said in his red book that such changes could sometimes assume an independent nature and so might persist even after carbohydrates had been curtailed. He did not say, I noticed, that it was therefore not worth trying, just that this may limit or delay success in, say, slimming.

But back to carbohydrate overload. One thing I couldn't figure out was the bit about the 'working compromise'. It was fine for No. 1 and No.2 to swap places two hours or so after a meal and if we ate carbohydrates modestly, yes, the working compromise would work. But even if we ate sweet and stodgy things all day and so blocked access to fat all day, surely there were still eight hours or so left during the night for Controller No.2 to get busy? I asked Uncle, who said something about bodies getting into a habitual way of doing things and that, if things had got that bad, eight hours weren't long enough to make the switch to a different fuel. He then painted a gruesome picture of us consuming protein from our own body tissues to provide the necessary sugar and there was something even more gruesome about plugging the gaps in the damaged tissues with fat. It sounded dire. I searched in my books but, except in cases of real starvation, I could not find out what 'that bad' meant in practice and how much carbohydrate it would take to get there.

Talking of 'things getting that bad', surely it was not just the controllers that could get cantankerous: think for a moment of the poor cells! I knew that millions if not trillions of our cells stored minute amounts of starch, fat and protein to provide energy, and that they didn't want much sugar in the first place. You can imagine how, when asked to take in ever more sugar, there has to come a time when the cells are full to the gunwales of sugar and say 'enough is enough': they sulk, resist the commands from outside (defying Controller No.1) and shut their gates. Cells would have to have been very provoked over a long period of time to behave like that, I thought.

As for cantankerous controllers, imagine being a guard and permanently called out on emergency duty, for this was the sort of situation that, in effect, our controllers were in when we lived with too much carbohydrate in our diet. True, No.1's job was to be always on duty, always present in the bloodstream and to be around after each mealtime as well as getting on happily with other tasks. That was fine and normal. No.1 obligingly saw to the odd bit of excess sugar now and then, or even several times a day, without making too much fuss, but always on emergency duty? That was a different kettle of fish. It was too much to demand and definitely too much to be sustained. What had Uncle said? 'No time off: too busy dealing with the problem of sugar!'

So then what? Increasing the size of the guard does not long suffice. Over-demanded Controller No.1 starts thinking 'I know what is coming – my owner always has toast and marmalade for breakfast and she has sugar with her coffee and there will be constant other carbohydrates coming in throughout the day, and evening, too – so forget all this fine tuning, I'll just throw out a generous handful of instructions as to removing sugar from the bloodstream: it's sure to cover the need.' Cover the need it does, but proves over-generous and too many instructions are sent out.

The result of this largesse is that too much sugar is removed from the bloodstream and the owner feels wobbly, anxious and irritable. Soon other controllers from the sugar squad rush in to help and they do a good job. These are Controller No.1's opposite number and the 'fight or flight' controllers which between them see to the topping up of the sugar level again: they initiate feelings of hunger and order the creating and mobilising of sugar from within the body. But the 'generous handful' of No.1 has become habitual and these controllers, too, become over-worked. The owner now feels as though she were living on a roller coaster. Not good, not good at all.

So this was why, when I wanted to eat again half an hour after a meal, Uncle had accused me of having false hunger? My 'hunger' was real in the sense of the blood's immediate need for sugar, but this was the consequence, not of having too little to eat, but rather of my having had too much of, well, need I say what? It's true I felt wobbly and also irritable, sometimes fearful, sometimes tearful. Eating a sweetie would put that right for a while, until the next time, that is. And it was always difficult to stop eating biscuits. I would take one and then find I had finished the whole packet. It was the same with chocolate. Oh dear!

I began to see something of what Uncle was driving at when I had formerly quizzed him about excess carbohydrate and he had summed it up in the one word: 'trouble'. I delved back into my red book. Apparently, if this condition lasts too long, Controller No.1 gradually becomes exhausted and can't hack it any more: fewer and fewer instructions are sent out and so sugar mounts in the bloodstream unchecked. The owner now has a recognised ailment. Uncle said that, at this stage, it was often still possible to live safely and healthily by keeping to his diet. This he knew from long experience as a doctor.

It did make sense, I thought. If you ate few enough carbohydrates, this had to mean no excess sugar in the blood. Then there would no longer be any call on Controller No.1

for emergency duty, no longer any reason for the cells to go on strike. Rather than giving drugs to force the cells to open their gates to take in even more sugar, Uncle's diet offered cells a fuel more suited to the purpose. I could imagine how gratefully No.1 would return to regular duties only, now that overtime was not necessary. Might this stop all those ill effects from all those disturbances in all those different parts of the body and in the future, too, I wondered?

Yet if the overload of carbohydrate continues and so the need for overtime, the person in question has to be supplied with a stand-in from outside to assist her own over-wearied controller. She then feels better in herself and can carry on eating as before. But – and this is a big but – if she does not mend her ways and reduce her sugars and starches, this does not stop the cells eventually resisting, nor does it prevent the other controllers being adversely effected, and particularly No.2, so important for tissue quality. Result: all sorts of other trouble, some very serious and much of it avoidable! Good old Uncle Wolfi, he must have saved his patients from so much suffering. I was proud of him.

I told Mum of all I had read and she became very serious, then said: "Well, you have to hand it to the old boy!"

"What, my chocolate?" I said, alarmed.

"No, silly, can't you see he's trying, after his own fashion, to give you a wake-up call?"

"I . . . um . . . well . . . but . . ." is all I could manage.

I looked at Mum, but Mum, lapsing into deep thought, just muttered: "I wonder, I just wonder."

'DOING A WOLFI'

Mum and I did a lot of wondering. About a week later we were having a meal together and were reflecting on Uncle Wolfi's last visit.

"I thought Uncle was very considerate in not bogging us down with the long names of all those internal bits and pieces. I've got enough to learn at school," I grumbled, adding, "and I was thankful he didn't talk about all those awful ailments which he seems to treat so successfully. There were more than enough in his book."

"You mean those he so charmingly refers to as the 'civilisatory diseases'?"

"Yes, and Mum, you ought to have another look at the red book – the list is awesome!"

"I wish you would not use that term, dear!"

"Oh, Mum, but it does seem Uncle has found a wonderful tool for healing, don't you think?"

"I believe so," she said, "judging by my own very limited experience, anyway. Praise be, we do not need him to treat us for any of his 'awful ailments', as you call them." Not yet, I thought inwardly. "But perhaps proper instructions as to his diet . . . we do require," she added.

I looked at Mum. What did she mean by 'we do require'? Had she made up her mind? Would she take the plunge?

"I could give Uncle a ring and ask his advice, maybe," I said cautiously.

"No, I'll give the old boy a bell myself." She called him 'the old boy' as often as he called me Sparrow. "I think we should give it a try," said Mum mildly. She looked at me: "don't you agree?"

"I suppose I agree," I said, heavy-hearted. I had visions of all sorts of goodies disappearing from the shelves of the fridge and a bleak freezer stocked with reindeer meat. "Yes, Mum, if Uncle says I ought, I'll give it a go."

Uncle was duly phoned. The feedback I got was that he was delighted and wished us every success with it; as Mum was 'of a certain age' it would be better for her to start slowly, say take three months in cutting down to his magic amount, but that I could probably cut down straight away.

"You don't think I'm going to sit here fiddling with my fish fingers while you scoff all the chips do you?" I said, testily.

"The old boy did suggest it was always easier if another member of the household was also doing it – and at the same rate – he said it preserved domestic harmony!" she smiled, knowingly. I grimaced, but Mum ignored me and went on: "And I was to make sure I did not cut down fat as well as carbohydrate which, he said, was where a lot of people went wrong. I told him to have no fear – it would be a blessed relief not to have to worry any more about eating fat. I said I was already eating a little more fat and that some days I found I wanted more than others. He said that was how it should be and that, provided you chose natural fats and cut down the carbohydrates enough, the body regulated its own appetite for them

117

– too little and you wanted more, too much and you felt nauseous."

"Uncle is right," I put in, "you couldn't eat a whole packet of butter in one go, could you!" I smiled at my own cleverness, and added: "But if the meat is dry, a little butter is good." I had seen Uncle Wolfi do this.

"The good news," said Mum, "is that on this diet the need for calories also regulates itself, so we can throw out altogether any thought of counting calories – a red herring, according to your Uncle. Oh, and he said it would 'do the little one good'. Little one! I could learn to drive in a couple of years: I was almost adult, though I admit I was not feeling like one at that moment. "But that first we needed to do a little homework." Not more homework, surely!

However, this preparatory work was fun. During this couple of weeks, we were to eat exactly as we usually did, but first we needed to acquire kitchen scales that weighed in grams. Mum only had the old-fashioned sort with a big brass pan and massive weights for measuring pounds of damsons, plums and sugar in the autumn when we made jam, but somewhere in the attic I'm sure I had seen an even older pair of scales – the sort apothecaries of old used for weighing out their potions by the gram. It had an upright pole and a balancing arm with a small brass pan hanging from either end. I had liked the box of tiny weights you put in one pan to get it level with what you were weighing in the other. Yes, that would do for now.

By doing lots of weighing and measuring, we were to get to know the amount of carbohydrate we were accustomed to eat. I was glad that Uncle Wolfi had sent us two little charts to make this easier, as I could never make any sense of the 'nutritional information' on food packets and, in any case, fresh fruit didn't usually have labels.

The theory may be OK," I said, wavering a little in my resolve, "but to actually do it?" I eyed the fruit bowl piled high with oranges, bananas and kiwis. "Here we are thinking of cutting carbohydrates, when fruit is supposed to be so good for us that we are to eat it many times a day."

"If you ask me – which I know you don't often choose to – I say there's a right muddle over it all." said Mum. "They tell us to eat mostly carbohydrates, and starches are fine but not if those starches are white and refined. My gran ate white bread and lived until she was 93 in good health; mind you, she didn't eat much of anything."

"Did I tell you, Mum, how one day in class I asked our teacher whether sugar wasn't to be found in all those pieces of fruit we are told to eat daily? She said yes and no! Fruit contained sugars, yes, but not sugar; that we were to avoid sugar, especially if was white, not though other sugars, which we were to eat freely. All round the classroom shoulders had shrugged, signalling that we neither understood nor intended to obey."

I could laugh as I thought of this now, but not so when I worked out one third of Uncle Wolfi's daily prescription and then weighed out the requisite amount of breakfast cereal in grams and saw how small the portion was. "I could eat a day's worth of carbohydrate for breakfast alone," I complained.

"We clearly have some unlearning to do," said Mum, smiling. "Above all, if we are really going to 'do a Wolfi', we must allow ourselves to be guided by him. The old boy, after all, has had nearly fifty years' experience with this way of eating and he is very sensitive to the well-being of his patients: he would be the first to draw a halt if he thought he had got it wrong about his medical advice. He told me the other day that seriously ill patients should be under a doctor's guidance and that, for such patients, he himself reduced carbohydrate very gradually and in stages, pausing at each stage until he was sure it was safe enough for them to proceed. And there are some medical conditions your Uncle wouldn't think of dieting. So none of your talking of 'magic amounts' to your Great-Aunt Hilda, as though she could just 'do a Wolfi' all of a sudden and all would be well." Aunt Hilda was old, quite poorly and often bed-ridden. Mum paused to give time for this to sink in.

"In the 1970's, there was this American doctor," she continued, "whom your Uncle thought was cutting people's carbohydrate both far too much and too rapidly, and he flew all the way to America to warn him of the dangers – I bet you didn't know that!"

"Did the American doctor listen to Uncle?" I wondered.

"I don't for a moment think so. It certainly did not change his advice to people, but that is not the point, is it?"

"You mean Uncle Wolfi had done his responsible bit?"

"Quite! Anyway, we might be a bit tired at first, but not if we take it slowly enough and we are to shout if we come across or suspect any hitches. Yes, until we have both been long enough on the diet to be able to judge for ourselves what works best for us, we must trust to his experience and guidance."

Mum now thought of a practical way forward. We would take two sheets of paper and put them up on the kitchen wall; on each we would draw a big food hamper. In the first, from which we could freely help ourselves without feeling that someone was looking over our shoulder, we would put the permitted food. Knowing how Uncle thought, we were not surprised that, apart from honey, he more or less allowed us free choice of any kind of food from the animal kingdom: fish, poultry or meat (the lean and the fat), eggs and animal fats such as lard and suet. Steak and kidney pudding with real suet – heavenly! (Just a minute: the flour in the crust would have to go in the next basket.) We could have Uncle's notion of the best of dairy foods: cheese, fresh cream, butter and ghee ad lib (but not low-fat cheese or milk, not in this basket anyway). Vegetable oils were also permitted, though not preferred. Uncle also gave a free hand with what he calls watery salad vegetables, in other words those without much substance to them such as lettuce, tomatoes, cucumber etc, also the leafy sort of vegetables, together with olives, mushrooms and courgettes; he said their carbohydrates scarcely counted.

"Couldn't you just live happily on such a picnic basket?" sighed Mum.

In the second, we would put all foods containing any appreciable amount of carbohydrate. Uncle's table included, in descending order from highest to lowest: sugar; honey; cereals; dried fruit; bread; beans and lentils; potatoes, bananas, sweetcorn and nuts; sweet fruit such as apples or pears; fresh or frozen peas and so on through various vegetables to yoghurt and milk. Of course, the carbohydrate content of all those ready-prepared foods we ate, like pizza and pies, also had to be counted, but the labels would help. Sugary drinks must also go on the list. Uncle thought fruit juice best diluted and that even small glasses still counted, as did sweets and chocolate. Come to think of it, this was the basket we did mostly live from. There was big change afoot!

"I think 'carbs', 'carbos' and 'carbohydrates' are all ugly words, whichever way you say them," said Mum. "It reminds me of chemistry lessons! I vote we stick to 'sugars and starches', don't' you?"

"Not easy," I replied sagely. "To 'do a Wolfi' properly, we have to learn about quantities, so we can't escape the word entirely."

"A great pity, such horrid words and at mealtimes, too," rejoined Mum.

"There is a way," I announced, remembering Uncle's tales of his time in Vienna. "Luckily for us, Uncle has a wonderfully simple way of calculating. He uses bread units. All you have to do is to count 12 grams of carbohydrate to each bread unit: et voila! Well, he actually said 12 grams of available carbohydrate, by which he didn't mean the total carbohydrate in any one food, but rather the amount the body could extract from the food for use. So now you know!"

"Come to think of it, doesn't one of his charts use bread units?" commented Mum.

"I must read them", I said, feeling a little guilty that I had not done so. "All I know is that our eventual goal is to be six bread units a day each. But slowly, slowly, catch a monkey! What do you say, Mum?"

We had three months – or as long as we chose – to get

used to a new balance in the way we selected items of food. There was time enough but, using Uncle's charts, we would make a start. So we set about with a will, doing all the weighing and measuring of all the items of food that we normally ate. Mum and I worked out that our usual consumption of carbohydrate probably averaged about 30 bread units a day. It was a far cry from six – and I didn't admit to the sweeties! We then spent time working out what a bread unit actually looked like on the plate. We had giggled when we first shared a medium-sized banana between us, as it seemed so stingy; it did, though, represent one bread unit for each of us and from then on we had that picture in our minds. Likewise one egg-sized potato was the equivalent of one bread unit, as was one tablespoon of cooked rice, two dates, one medium apple or one medium slice of bread.

In this way, we gradually assembled a mental picture gallery of one bread unit's worth of all the foods we normally ate. As a reference point, Uncle Wolfi's table of equivalence definitely had to have a place on the kitchen wall to keep jogging our memories as to how much we could allow ourselves to take from the second hamper on any one day.

I needn't have worried about the content of the fridge. At first, it stayed the same. Then, very gradually, I noticed a few changes but they were not disagreeable ones. There was some new fruit juice 'with no added sugar' that I hadn't tried before. There were different cheeses and some pâté, and sometimes a lovely big egg and ham flan with very thin pastry. There might be a packet of some very tempting-looking vine tomatoes that smelt like the real thing. I wondered where Mum was now doing the shopping! And there was more besides, with lots of variety. Then it turned out that Uncle had said she should not just cut down on the sugars and starches but was to make sure there were attractive alternatives always available and ones that would provide the right sort of nourishment both for her and for a growing lass.

Probably the biggest change was that Mum started doing much more of her own cooking and got me involved whenever she could. Packets, tins and many ready-made foods were less and less to be found in our house and I would often get a waft of a delicious stew as I came down our drive on the way back from school. That was definitely a plus! Moreover, since the change was to be slow, at first we ate two potatoes instead of three or four, or we took only two slices of toast with our more traditional breakfast. Previously we had chomped through the best part of a loaf between us, both of us being somewhat addicted to toast, especially with the additions of jam, honey or marmalade. Experimentally, we allowed ourselves only a smidgeon of marmalade and found that, with a little extra butter, this was tasty enough. One day it might be only one slice of toast, but there was no hurry.

The thought of marmalade took me back to the old days and my holidays by the lake, and Uncle helping himself at breakfast time to a spoonful of marmalade with his cream – and without any toast at all! But then he was not a bread sort of man. I remembered how he had proclaimed happily that, except for what I now thought of as his 'important proviso', as long as it suited them, people could eat whatever they liked on his diet. He said that he was only strict about what really mattered and that his patients were more satisfied and likely to persevere longer with the diet if they had maximum choice as to what was on their plate. On that occasion, Uncle Wolfi had looked straight at me: "Of course, I do trust people to have some common sense!" Had he expected me to want all my daily carbohydrate from peppermint creams? And all in one go?

I now learnt that Uncle Wolfi had warned Mum to see to it that I ate very regularly, dividing my carbohydrates fairly evenly over the three main meals. If at first I needed to take the edge off between meals, I was to have appropriate snacks to hand. I will say she was very good about this and I'm sure it helped. She would provide me with a small packet of nuts, cold sausage or a piece of cheese and, if she thought I couldn't otherwise avoid biscuits, she would supply me with nuts and raisins or a small packet of crisps. Something about the lesser of evils! Neither of us had yet tried the snack of putting unsalted butter on a piece of cheese, which Uncle had done when he first cut down on carbohydrate.

Somehow, just by taking a little less of things on the rationed list and by playing bread unit games, we managed to cut down to twenty units within a month. Mum gave up sugar and milk in her coffee, for instance, and had rediscovered the delight of pouring cream on the top of fresh black coffee and drinking the coffee through it. She said it reminded her of the cafés of her youth and I loved to see her taking such pleasure in something so simple. She felt fine so far and was minded to continue.

In our attempt to 'do a Wolfi' – well, to start doing the

diet – as well as of potatoes, we had both taken slightly smaller helpings of rice and pasta and eaten more of the beans, meat, cheese or egg that accompanied such food. For breakfast, if we didn't have bacon and egg, I ate beans on toast and Mum might have a cheese and tomato sandwich or yoghurt with a few prunes. Strange to say, neither of us felt hungrier for eating less. To be honest, at this stage we scarcely noticed the reduction of bread units.

In another month, we had reached twelve bread units. Mum had lost a few pounds and was looking good; she said felt she could stay on that amount of carbohydrate forever. I think she only reduced further for my sake, as I still had the occasional wobble. So we persevered and were getting the hang of it. Instead of bananas, for instance, I got to love savoury 'fillers' like humous on crispbread or oatcake.

We had found that eating some fat with each meal – whether using olive oil in the salad dressing, tossing our veg in coconut oil or bacon fat instead of cooking them with water or using the meat fat in the gravy or in soup – somehow sustained us and stopped us hankering after carbohydrates. We were still eating less overall and we didn't feel that we were eating any more fat than before: it was difficult to know. As we were eating less packaged foods, we certainly ate less 'hidden' fat and less commercially changed fats.

I was beginning to feel more peaceful in myself and less excitable. However, despite being quite well behaved in general, my progress was not uneventful.

One Saturday, after a good breakfast and a tiny protein-rich snack mid-morning, I was feeling fine and quite complacent. In a snack bar with friends, I ordered for lunch a baked potato with tuna mayonnaise. When it came to the table, it was the most whopping great potato I had ever seen: at a rough estimate it must have been at least eight bread units worth. Naturally I ate the whole lot with my old gusto – I think it was my eyes that so tempted me, not my appetite – and I felt not a little full. Within the hour, that old unbearable feeling of faintness mixed with desperate need for more food came upon me and I found myself suggesting ice-cream to my friends, who were eager enough. By the time I got home, some two hours and two chocolate bars later, I was extremely crochety and immediately burst into a flood of tears.

Later that day, I phoned Uncle. But when I had told him how I was no saint and confessed what had happened, he was not put out at all. I could almost feel goodwill being beamed down the phone.

"Sparrow," he said, "none of us can be a saint until after we are dead, so enjoy being a fallible human: forgive yourself and try again!" It was sage advice. So I did forgive myself and did try again. No more spaghetti on toast, no more pasta with garlic bread and cake to follow. Gradually it got easier not to overdo things, to choose a café where they did small platefuls or to take, say, just a small piece of cake at a friend's party or a small helping of fruit juice. That way I could join in the fun but keep my system stable for I knew, though I didn't tell anyone, that Uncle was helping me to stop upsetting my controllers and so, if possible, to avoid real trouble in the future.

LAST VISIT

The following winter saw a second visit from Uncle Wolfi. It was late October and he wasn't long back from Austria.

"What lovely warm hands you have, Sparrow" he said, as he took my hands and kissed me on both cheeks. Warm feet, too, I thought, gratified that my progress showed. Mum, too, looked glad that Uncle had noticed.

"Thank you. We had a good journey back to England and just beat the winter snows," he said, as he sat down to our evening meal. Uncle Wolfi tucked heartily into the roast lamb, took plenty of the gravy and one small roast potato, politely declining the mint sauce and cabbage cooked with caraway seeds.

"Don't you like my vegetables?" I asked, a little hurt as I was getting to be proud of my newly acquired art of cooking them.

"Thank you, but personally I do not often eat vegetables. I tend to see plant food as an optional extra, but please feel free to enjoy them yourself." I was pleased when he accepted the dainty dish of fruit salad that I had prepared for him and then helped himself to more cream. "It worries my wife, so she puts a small glass of vegetable juice by my plate, which I dutifully drink!" he said, with the old twinkle in his eyes.

Uncle had aged since we last saw him. He was distinctly

frailer and a little slower, his walks were shorter, bedtime a little earlier and, since receiving an infected tick bite walking in the woods near his home in Austria, one of his hips was now plaguing him. But Uncle Wolfi was still upright and he still preserved his air of distinction. His lovable mixture of serious concern and realism was still apparent and his irrepressible humour and sense of irony seemed to keep him calm and unflustered as he got older.

We sat down round the bright fire and he looked us up and down approvingly. "Na, und?" he asked, this time meaning 'how are you both and what have you been up to', whilst his approving glance meant 'I see the diet is having its effect.'

"I think we are quite converts!" said Mum.

"But I am not offering a religion!" said Uncle Wolfi, laughing. "And you, Sparrow, my special secretary? I was very happy with the last letter you helped me with: thank you." I looked bashfully at the floor, pleased he was pleased. "And many people liked the summary of my main book that we did together. I still can't work out how you are gaining such insight into my work but, at my club, my colleagues joke that at last they understand what I am going on about! But where are your hundreds of questions?"

"I am struggling with GIs," I confessed, glad of a change of subject.

Mum laughed. "When your gran was at school, GIs were what all the girls dreamed of, if only for the illicit cigarettes and the silk stockings."

"GIs?" asked Uncle looking puzzled.

"Yes, all that about complex carbohydrates being slowly absorbed. It looks like your own teaching has been superseded." I explained.

"Ah," said Uncle nodding, but not without one of his special smiles. "Anything else?"

At this point, Mum disappeared on the pretext of doing the dishes.

"Actually, Uncle Wolfi," I said quietly, "Mum is going through what she calls 'the change' and since she's cut right down, she says all signs of it have completely disappeared."

"Good, good," he said. "I have many female patients who are very happy with the changes this way of eating brings." I am not sure he had understood me about Mum, but it didn't matter. "And about vegetables, some of my patients do not tolerate them very well – my GI patients, that is."

"Touché! Uncle," I said approvingly.

"Yes, my gut patients are not always thankful for certain vegetables nor, for that matter, are they always grateful for wholemeal bread and cereals."

"I read somewhere that fibre can hinder the absorption of nutrients," I commented.

"Not only that, but it can also speed the passage through the digestive tract. To some people this can, of course, be of help, but many of my patients find things go through them too quickly already and so need to avoid such rough things for some time, sometimes for life. And it does them good to do so. I have letters from patients who had had very serious bowel troubles and who have been free for thirty or forty years by cutting down on carbohydrate and keeping wholemeal bread to a minimum, sometimes avoiding it altogether."

"It takes guts to stick to a diet that long," I said, awed at the prospect.

"It helps the guts, certainly," countered Uncle with a

knowing smile. "But, you know, it is best not to think of it as a diet, more a natural way of eating. Then any time-span is OK."

This mention of a natural way of eating gave me a nostalgic pang for my old way of eating, which I had assumed natural in those days. I asked as casually as I could: "In general, though, Uncle, when can people put the carbos back in again?" I had adopted this word so distasteful to Mum.

"If you mean when can people resume the excesses that caused them to be ill in the first place . . ."

"Well, I know that would be stupid," I interrupted somewhat sheepishly, as I had known full well what Uncle would reply. "What I mean is, once people are properly better, can they put up their carbohydrates a little?"

"Reports from my patients vary in this matter: some find they can eventually eat a little more carbohydrate and stay well, others have to remain on a low level in the long-term. Once used to it, it is not arduous. Our bodies and our health tend to guide us and warn us with a nudge of our old troubles when we overdo things too much or too often."

Mum returned with a glass of wine for herself and for Uncle Wolfi. This he gratefully accepted, and we all three settled down for a long chat about the happenings of the intervening year.

"It is not as though we used to eat much junk food anyway and I always provided wholemeal bread," said Mum at one point, "but since we cut down to six bread units, which was over six months ago, I must say that that lass over there," she indicated me with a gesture of her head, "has been a lot easier to live with!"

"My point entirely!"

"Thanks, both of you!" I said not very graciously, but Uncle ignored it.

"It is true that a wholefood diet with its so-called fibre-rich complex carbohydrates will fill you up more than refined foods do. Therefore people may find they eat less carbohydrate anyway," said he.

"Well, cutting right down, whole or no, helped my wobbles," I confessed.

"In such cases," said Uncle, and I was grateful he made it impersonal, "it is essential to cut down carbohydrate from all sources to the level that stabilises the blood sugar mechanism – which I usually found to be about six or seven bread units, sometimes a little less."

"You mean, cut down to a level that stops provoking all those overworked controllers and gives them a well-earned rest?" I said, teasing him a little. He nodded, lapsing into thought. "It must save on a lot of drugs," I muttered to myself.

"Naturally, the effect depends partly on the level of carbohydrate consumed," Uncle observed after a time, his eyes on the tapping thumbs of his clasped hands. "But, you see, directly or indirectly, all the major controllers are involved in dealing with carbohydrate overload and are therefore affected by it; this of course can be detrimental to our health in so many ways." I was glad I had got this bit right. "How much, in what way and how soon our health is disturbed depends on a number of factors, such as age, level of physical activity, strength of constitution, hereditary predisposition and so on, as I think I mentioned."

I shook my head slowly in dismay: "I don't stand a chance then really," I said, thinking of my wider family.

"Of course you do! How many times must I tell you that predisposition does not equate to destiny: predisposition still gives you a chance and you, Sparrow, are already taking the right way forward. My point was to give you an idea why such a surprisingly wide range of medical conditions are aggravated by an excess of carbohydrates and so may respond favourably to sufficient carbohydrate restriction."

He looked up at me: "And yes, it does save on drugs. A fragmentary approach can lead to the use of many different drugs whereas, by this simple dietary measure alone, a whole cluster of raised regulatory activity can be lowered and restored to normal."

"You mean the body is capable of its own micromanagement and we don't need to do it by giving all those drugs?"

"I mean that perhaps there would be less need for such measures if . . ."

"If we had more respect for the cuisine of our ancient relatives?" I suggested.

"Quite so," agreed Uncle, smiling at the thought.

"Don't you give your patients drugs, then Uncle?" I ventured to ask.

"While their bodies are adjusting to this new way of eating, patients with particularly severe medical conditions, even when carbohydrates are reduced very, very slowly, often still need help over the transition time: low level dosage of medication for a few months usually suffices. In certain circumstances or in cases where I feel the diet to be insufficient on its own to bring about the requisite healing, I may have to recommend surgery. I use both drugs and surgery as little as possible."

"Uncle, you just mentioned the word 'normal': restoring to normal a whole lot of disturbed regulatory activity, I think you said. In your red book, you talk of all sorts of blood levels normalising and of all sorts of organs being a lot happier. Do you think that the key to your success is that in some way or other the diet itself brings things in general back to normal?"

"Naturally, we are not sure these days what 'normal' is," said Uncle Wolfi both modestly and quite seriously. "It is some time since the Ice Age! What I can say for certain is that my diet tends to bring things within the parameters that modern medicine recognises as normal."

"Well, both Mum and I feel the better for it," I said appreciatively.

"I'm very glad of it."

"So our controllers are co-operating again as they should and harmony prevails?" I added.

"Quite so," said Uncle.

And harmony did prevail that evening.

"Uncle Wolfi, I was reading that book you wrote with your veterinary friend, the professor. We don't do biochemistry at school so most of it was over my head, but there was one statement that quite blew my mind. Your professor said that eating excess carbohydrate adversely affected the internal regulation of all warm-blooded animals. Can that be true? All warm-blooded animals?"

"Personally, I can only speak for humans, and perhaps hens," he replied in his ironic way. "My professor, as you call him, has much wider research experience. Remember we do share a lot of our body processes with the other animals, you know," added Uncle Wolfi with a chuckle.

"But they give cows molasses and treat horses to sugar lumps!" I rejoined, worrying if this counted as excess and thinking back to what Uncle had explained to me about my neighbour's blackbirds and their raisins years ago. "And I read that they feed sugar to cows because they want to change the quality of the fats in the cow's milk to make it good for us."

"It seems, having lost respect for the wisdom of nature's laws, we are losing our way," remarked Uncle sadly.

"There was another point in that book that I wanted to ask you about," I said. "Stress, you said, was essential to life – in the right amount, that is – and you said that, in modern life, there were three main sources of excessive stress: namely a relative lack of exercise, mental and emotional stress and carbohydrates. If I understood correctly, both of you agreed that if people reduced the stress of excess carbohydrate, the other two stresses would be less, well, less stressful. Is that what you still think, Uncle Wolfi?"

"That book was years ago, Sparrow, and perhaps we should add environmental pollution of various sorts. But yes, I still think carbohydrates a stress and a major one at that. When excess carbohydrate was removed from their diet, I found with my patients that a great many body systems did calm down, and this included the nervous system. Reduction of stress also showed itself in that bones and muscles, even internal muscles like the heart, tended to improve and external muscles tended to tone up without special exercise. Less stress? Perhaps that is it," he said humbly.

"Oh Uncle, I really think you should be famous!" I said quite sincerely.

"Well, they haven't exactly given me a knighthood but, after what seems like a lifetime of swimming against the tide, I am beginning to get a modicum of recognition. But you know, it doesn't work like that. Just because you find something to be true – and you can show it in practice – does not necessarily dismantle a myth."

"You mean, for example, that finding something isn't so is not enough to correct a belief that it is so? But, Uncle Wolfi . . ." I added in naïve protest.

"Oh, I found that out long ago, Sparrow. Let me tell you a little story about the war-time," he said, settling himself more comfortably in his armchair. "I was working on a way to save the lives of pilots in high-flying aircraft. Cabins were already pressurised but if for any reason this pressure failed at very high altitudes the pilots lost consciousness, which obviously was not propitious. It was thought at the time that this loss of consciousness was caused by bubbles arising in the blood vessels from the change in pressure. However, I was able to show that the bubbles only came later and that consciousness was lost immediately the pressure failed, giving the pilots no time to take remedial action. My discovery enabled me to design a suit, which automatically inflated the instant pressure dropped. It was a short-acting device, such as is seen nowadays on astronauts working outside the space shuttle, only the oxygen flask was worn on the leg. It was my prototype of the space suit, which I think you know about. Yet here we are half a century later and I still read that it is bubbles that cause loss of consciousness. The folklore of science is so difficult to shift!"

Uncle was gazing into the dying fire, slowly shaking his head as he thought of this.

"Perhaps it is the same with the work I did subsequently on carbohydrates? So strong is the belief that carbohydrates should predominate in our diet that my findings about the harmful effects of overload do not dent modern nutritional folklore. Plus ça change!" he said, shrugging his shoulders. Then, spreading out his hands, Uncle added his familiar, "Na ja, na ja! Yes, perhaps demonstration of a truth is seldom enough and the correction of belief trails years behind." Uncle Wolfi seemed accepting of this statement of how things operate but, in reality, I knew that he had never given up hope of publishing a definitive paper that would open the eyes, if not of the world, then at least of the medical profession, that it might abandon what Uncle saw as its erroneous thinking and find its rightful path once again.

PROMISE

It was the last time I saw Uncle Wolfi, but we by no means lost touch with one another. When I was quite a bit younger, I had written a story simply called 'Uncle Wolfi' to tease him. When he eventually got round to reading it – his desk was always piled high with papers and journals that must have been far more pressing for his attention – Uncle had phoned me to say how much he and Helen had enjoyed reading the story together. His only comment was that I had made him out to be a far nicer person than he really was. So I had now made him, at times, a little over-bearing, occasionally snapping at his 'little Sparrow'. I also added in a lot of what I had since learnt.

After his last visit, Uncle had taken this new attempt away with him to read on the train. A few weeks later he rang me: "Sparrow, I like what you have written a great deal and I especially admire your fanciful imagination."

"Poetic license," I answered in excuse.

"That is all very well, Sparrow, but from this point on, I feel it would be best if I tell my own story," said Uncle decisively. "I would like to do this in English so, of course, I shall still need help with that."

"I did my best," I protested. Then I relented, as I knew I had had great fun writing the stories: "What would you like me to do then, Uncle?"

Uncle Wolfi considered for a moment, then said: "I suggest I tell my story to you and you write it down for me."

"We could call it: Who's afraid of the big bad wolf?" I said, my imagination already running overtime. "You would be amazed at how many people feel threatened by the idea of 'cutting the carbs', as they put it. I know many of my classmates are afraid to even try."

"I will be amazed? You forget, Sparrow, that I have been helping people do just that for decades. I repeat: I, myself, will tell the story and you will confine yourself to writing it down in good English. Agreed? If you like, you can add to what I say from my books and articles or from what we have already discussed together, but you must show me every word you write – every word!"

"Oh, Uncle," I said, dithering a little. Then a thought struck me and I added eagerly: "I know, I could interview you. I am old enough now to be working for a local newspaper. Yes, I'll pretend to be a reporter."

"No Sparrow, no more of your pretending games – this is for real."

"You have made yourself quite clear, Uncle," I said, noting his firmness of purpose.

By this time, Uncle, too, had relented: "You've written a good story and I enjoyed it. In its way, I suppose what you say is sound."

"Albeit a product of my 'fanciful imagination', my story is our story – about you and me, Uncle Wolfi, and the special times we spent together. I would like to do something with it. I did learn so much from the conversations I had with you. They helped me get well and may help others to do likewise?" I suggested hopefully.

"I suppose such whimsical writing has its place and could, I think, be useful background for people unfamiliar with such matters. Do as you please with it, Sparrow." It was as near as I was going to get to his blessing and I was thankful.

"But will you also write me my own story?" Uncle was again asking. "You can understand, can't you Sparrow that I want to record in English my own memories of how I came to realise the detrimental effect of an overload of carbohydrate – and that I want it to be my book and my story?" Recently, there had been a work in English on his medical work, but Uncle felt that he had not had enough say in the book, so I could understand that he did not want a whippersnapper like me with her own ideas getting in the way of his project. "Will you do it? My story?"

"Including your confessions?" I asked, somewhat cheekily.

"Yes, I know you will demand something of the sort from me," said Uncle laughing. "We will have to see about that! Na, und?"

"Hand on heart, Uncle Wolfi," I replied, "as best I can, I will be your most true and faithful scribe: honest I will."

And so it came about that I had another exciting commission to fulfil. Uncle had said long ago that one day I might tell his story and so it was to be, though it was to take me many years and I was almost through university before it was finished. I slowly put together fragments of a great many letters that Uncle wrote in answer to a great many of mine; I incorporated information gathered from old articles and books that Uncle had written, from our numerous phone conversations and from his endless reminiscences, some of which he had related on his visits to us up North. I remember sending him questionnaires for him to fill in to make sure I had understood what he had said, and then asking the same questions again to crosscheck the answers just like a proper researcher. I was neither Uncle's Spatz nor his Schatz then, I fear!

During this time, I was full of youthful argumentativeness and I came out with enough doubts and 'yes, buts' to try the patience of a saint let alone that of Uncle Wolfi. On the other hand, Uncle himself was getting ever older. Perhaps not surprisingly, there were misunderstandings galore, sometimes because of difficulties with language, sometimes because of errors in his typing when, at his great age, Uncle abandoned his old typewriter and bravely tried to conquer the complexities of the modern computer. At times, stormy disagreements raged and once Uncle said that next to his close friend, the veterinary professor, I was his fiercest critic; then, when that particular storm had abated, said that he appreciated this in me. Our tiffs and clashes were always made up in the end and, most of the time, we were very close and positive and made good progress.

We even dreamed together of a vast work, combining some of my own reading with Uncle Wolfi's actual experience and ideas; half of it got written before it was put aside in favour of something on a smaller scale. I got busy on the new project, but Uncle Wolfi's longing for that definitive article would keep returning and I, for my part, would stubbornly persist in wanting to carry on with the story of his journey of discovery. Eventually, both the article and our grand aspirations were distilled into a short tale describing what I hoped was the very essence of what the enquirer into his life and work needed most to hear – and it <u>was</u> Uncle Wolfi's own exciting story and Uncle <u>did</u> read every word. But Uncle was ageing and I was too inexperienced to launch it myself, as Uncle hoped I would at the time. So, much to our mutual regret, that particular result of our long co-operation did not see the light of day during Uncle's lifetime.

During the last few years of his life, Uncle Wolfi did receive recognition for his medical work and more than a modicum. Honours just seemed to come pouring in, but he stayed as unassuming and modest as always.

"I myself don't need honours", he said to me, "but I'm glad of it for the sake of my work."

On one occasion, Uncle Wolfi was guest of honour in recognition of a new title that was being conferred on him; when it came time for refreshments, this pioneering advocate of a life with little or no bread – what was he handed? Sandwiches! Uncle must have appreciated the irony, though he said not a word. With a quiet dignity, Uncle Wolfi discreetly removed the outer layers of the sandwiches and ate the ham that was in the middle, carefully wiping his fingers on his napkin!

Uncle went on occasionally seeing patients until well after he was ninety years old. During these last years, Uncle Wolfi and Aunt Helen continued to over-winter in London and spend their summers in Austria. I had my own life to lead, but Uncle and I still kept in regular touch by phone. He and I had our special way of communicating, born of long practice. He used to tease me, saying that I got 'under his skin' and that I knew what he was thinking even if he had not yet said anything about it.

It was in this way that Uncle and I were still able to hold meaningful communications even when he was on his ebb-tide: I would phone and tell Uncle what I was doing and I could tell by the precise timing of his laughter that he was understanding me. Towards the end, I phoned him and reassured him that I had every intention of bringing out his tale so that his message would be more accessible to English speakers and I could tell from the encouraging noises he made that he still wanted me to do so. There were sounds of contentment when I whispered down the phone: "I will do it, Uncle, I promise."

Old age was catching up with him and, having reached the grand age of ninety-seven, my remarkable Uncle Wolfi died during his summer stay in his native Austria.

But I shall be good health to you nevertheless.

That poem again! Oh Uncle, I shall always remember you with gratitude and affection. And, dear Uncle Wolfi, now that you have

shaken your white locks at the runaway sun

perhaps it is time for your little Sparrow, in her own small way, to

sound

your precious secret

over the roofs of the world?

I would like to thank my family and friends for their help and encouragement and Charlotte Cornforth for the cover painting.